W9-AYG-340

RESTORING
FLEXIBILITY

RESTORING FLEXIBILITY

A Gentle Yoga-Based Practice to Increase Mobility at Any Age

Andrea Gilats, PhD, RYT

Text copyright © 2015 Andrea Gilats. Photographs copyright © 2015 Rapt Productions except as noted below. Design and concept copyright © 2015 Ulysses Press and its licensors. All rights reserved. Any unauthorized duplication in whole or in part or dissemination of this edition by any means (including but not limited to photocopying, electronic devices, digital versions, and the internet) will be prosecuted to the fullest extent of the law.

Published in the United States by:
Ulysses Press
PO Box 3440
Berkeley, CA 94703
www.ulyssespress.com

ISBN: 978-1-61243-491-9
Library of Congress Control Number: 2015937567

Printed in the United States
10 9 8 7 6 5 4 3 2 1

Acquisitions: Casie Vogel
Managing editor: Claire Chun
Editor: Lily Chou
Proofreader: Lauren Harrison
Indexer: Sayre Van Young
Front cover/interior design and layout: what!design @ whatweb.com
Cover artwork: © Rapt Productions
Interior artwork: Rapt Productions except page 3 © Jacob Lund/shutterstock.com; page 19 © Pressmaster/shutterstock.com; page 42 © sciencepics/shutterstock.com (hamstring) and Sebastian Kaulitzki/shutterstock.com (psoas); page 83 © otnaydur/shutterstock.com; page 97 © Kudla/shutterstock.com
Models: Baxter Bell, Andrea Gilats, Toni Silver

Please Note: This book has been written and published strictly for informational purposes, and in no way should be used as a substitute for consultation with health care professionals. You should not consider educational material herein to be the practice of medicine or to replace consultation with a physician or other medical practitioner. The author and publisher are providing you with information in this work so that you can have the knowledge and can choose, at your own risk, to act on that knowledge. The author and publisher also urge all readers to be aware of their health status and to consult health care professionals before beginning any health program.

This book is independently authored and published. No sponsorship or endorsement of this book by, and no affiliation with, any trademarked brands or products mentioned or pictured is claimed or suggested. All trademarks that appear in this book belong to their respective owners and are used here for informational purposes only. The author and publisher encourage readers to patronize the quality brands and other products mentioned and pictured in this book.

CONTENTS

INTRODUCTION

In 2006, life handed me a double whammy. I was diagnosed with both emphysema and Crohn's disease. I had probably been living with these conditions for years, but because I had grieved so long and hard after the loss of my husband to cancer in 1998, I hadn't paid attention to the slow but relentless worsening of my symptoms. But the universe works in mysterious ways and, as luck would have it, in late 2007, I moved into a condominium building that had a fitness center next door to it. My 62-year-old body joined the gym, and I began working with a trainer twice a week. Shortly after I started strength training, my gym began offering a yoga class. I decided to give it a try.

From the moment I found yoga, I felt like a duck in water. What amazed me was that the negative stories I had been telling myself about my physical abilities seemed irrelevant when it came to yoga. I've never been particularly athletic; I've never been good at sports. Back then, I spent most of my day at my desk or in meetings and, in the evening, I turned into a couch potato. But yoga changed all that. After years of avoidance, I had finally found a way to restore my confidence in my physical abilities.

No matter when you come to yoga, you'll carry your body's history with you to the mat. There, to my surprise, I learned that my history didn't limit me at all, nor did my age or my diseases and conditions. I began to realize that yoga was something I could get better at through practice, so I stayed with it. After just a few weeks, I began to see and feel the positive changes in my body. I also found myself feeling more energetic—I actually began to enjoy moving! By restoring my flexibility, I regained the mobility I had lost through inactivity, and because I had become more agile, physical activity became a pleasure, not a chore. Even housework became easier!

As a yoga teacher with a checkered body history, I want to help ensure that the continuing story of your body is long and happy. The purpose of this book is to help you restore your flexibility so that you can increase your mobility, stay active and independent as you age, and live longer. To help you meet these goals, I offer a safe, age-appropriate, individually customizable approach to yoga-based exercise for those of you who've never tried yoga and those of you who've practiced yoga in the past and would like to reconnect with it. Done over four weeks, this 25-minute, twice-weekly program features gentle poses, practice sequences, and techniques to help you:

- improve your posture and spinal flexibility so you can avoid the need for a walker down the road.

- release tightness in your shoulder joints so you can move your arms freely and reach farther.

- relax the muscles in your torso so you can twist and turn easily while keeping your spine safe.

- mobilize your hip joints and the muscles that move them so you can comfortably lengthen and widen your stance and bend forward, backward, and sideways without aggravating your low back.

- lower yourself to the ground and get up again safely and confidently so you can improve your agility, enjoy greater total-body flexibility, and reduce your chances of falling.

As you move through your yoga flexibility program, you'll see that your range of motion—how far you can comfortably move each part of your body in any direction—is expanding. That's flexibility. You'll also discover that you're becoming better able to safely and easily change your body position. That's agility, flexibility's kissin' cousin. As your flexibility practice becomes a regular habit, I hope you'll find yourself wanting to move more. When all is said and done, it's regular, frequent movement that will keep you mobile and independent for many years to come, no matter your age when you start.

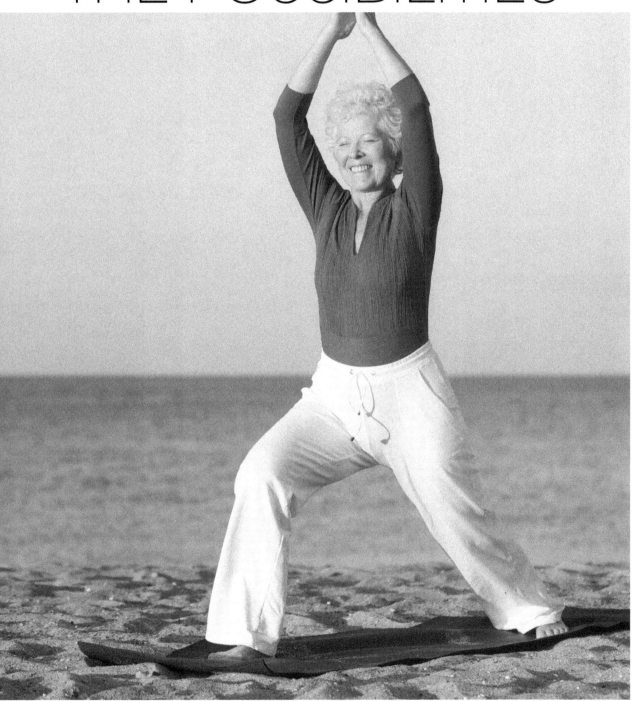

PART ONE

THE POSSIBILITIES

CHAPTER 1

WELCOME TO YOUR EXTRA-LONG LIFE

In his landmark 2008 book, *The Longevity Revolution*, renowned physician and gerontologist Robert Butler says that "from the Bronze Age to the end of the 19th century, life expectancy grew by only an estimated 29 years—from about 20 to about 50 years. But since the beginning of the 20th century in the industrialized world, there has been an unprecedented gain of more than 30 years of average life expectancy.... I call this unprecedented demographic transformation the Longevity Revolution."[1]

All of us reading this book are part of this transformation. We are—or will be—the lucky recipients of an ever-lengthening era of physical, intellectual, and social vitality after midlife. These extra years aren't tacked on to the ends of our lives—they come at a time when we're healthy enough to enjoy them. Thanks to modern medical advances like antibiotics and vaccines, this "bonus era" can last for two or three decades or more.

Better yet, the longer you've lived, the longer you're going to live. For example, if you're one of the 60 million Americans who have made it to age 60, odds are you're going to live another 20 to 30 years.[2] Our bonus years can be the best of our lives, but if we don't move our bodies regularly and frequently, we'll gradually lose our mobility and, with it, our ability to live independently. The bottom line? The longer we can preserve our mobility, the longer we'll live.

It's never too early or too late to take care of our future selves, especially when doing so can bring us joy in the present moment. When we fail to do the things today that will help ensure a longer, brighter succession of tomorrows, we aren't being fair to ourselves. We must make a point of getting up and moving today, otherwise we may not be able to get up and move tomorrow.

THE 70/30 PROPOSITION

We want to live long lives, and we also want to stay healthy for as long as possible. After all, a long life is only a gift if you feel good. The great news about healthy longevity is that our health span, including the number of years we can expect to enjoy good health later in life, is mostly in our own hands. Once you're past midlife, longevity is only about 30 percent genetic inheritance. The other 70 percent is related to lifestyle—how we take care of our bodies, how, where, and with whom we spend our time, and how we look at life.

Part of that 70 percent is as simple as taking our medicine. Today, medical advances have transformed life-threatening illnesses into manageable chronic conditions that allow us to live active, independent lifestyles throughout later life. In fact, many experts believe that as we age, well-being (an individual, subjective measure of how good we feel) may be a better indicator of overall health than the absence of disease.

Still, experts agree that sitting back and taking our medicine is probably not enough to significantly lengthen our health span. To help assure healthy longevity, we must also make positive lifestyle choices, such as eating nutritiously, connecting with people we care about and, most importantly, incorporating physical movement into our lives, both as part of our daily activities and through regular, planned exercise. This includes not only aerobic activities (like walking) for heart health, but also activities that keep our joints, muscles, and bones healthy. In fact, the American Heart Association has long recommended both aerobic exercise and twice-weekly flexibility training to help assure healthy longevity.[3]

CHAPTER 2

MOBILITY, FLEXIBILITY, & HEALTHY LONGEVITY

Mobility is the ability to move freely and easily. As long as we're mobile, we're free to live our lives the way we want. We can do what we want and go where we want. Physical independence also gives us the freedom to direct our own lives: make our own decisions, take care of ourselves, and participate in the adventures of life as fully as we wish. If we lose our physical mobility—even just some of it—we give up freedoms that we've counted on throughout our adult lives. We're used to counting on our bodies, but as our life journeys lengthen, we can no longer take physical mobility for granted.

The medical community characterizes physical mobility as the ability to climb stairs, walk a quarter of a mile over hill and dale, and respond to an emergency like a fire. Mobility is also measured by the distance we can travel from our homes without assistance, including that long-awaited vacation to our dream destination halfway around the world. Loss of mobility is not only inconvenient, frustrating, and depressing, it's associated with higher rates of disability, nursing home placement, and early mortality.[4]

Recent research has shown that the biggest risk factor for both mobility loss and early mortality in older adults is lack of physical activity,[5] but there's a flip side to this coin. Studies also show that taking up physical activity later in life not only lowers our risk of losing mobility, it adds years to our lives. This is not an all-or-nothing proposition—even light to moderate exercise is associated with higher odds of recovery for people who already have some loss of mobility.[6]

Joints and muscles need motion to stay healthy. The less we move, the tighter our joints and muscles become, and the tighter our joints and muscles become, the harder it is to move. Gradually, over time, we move less and less. The hard truth? Only by moving our bodies in all directions can the synovial fluids stored in the cavities of our joints wash over our cartilage, keeping our joints lubricated and in healthy working condition. Without healthy joints and muscles, we cannot preserve, let alone increase, our physical mobility.

THE FLEXIBILITY/LONGEVITY CONNECTION

Flexibility—the ability to safely and easily move our joints through their range of motion—is now considered a predictor of longevity. For years, researchers have pointed to a connection between flexibility and longevity but, more recently, that connection has been proven. In 2012, a breakthrough study showed that healthy levels of flexibility, along with sufficient strength and coordination (that's our friend, agility), was "remarkably predictive of all-cause mortality" among a group of 2000 people aged 51 to 80.[7]

The study was simple. Participants were asked to lower themselves to a seated position on the ground and get back up again using as little support from their hands, arms, or knees as they felt necessary. Using a 10-point scale to measure flexibility, researchers scored participants according to how much support they needed in order to lower and rise. Incredibly, just a one-point rise in the score correlated to a 21 percent reduction in mortality over the study's six-year follow-up period. This means that getting just a little better at coming down to the ground and getting up again can add years to our lives.[8]

WHY WE LOSE FLEXIBILITY AS WE AGE

There's no denying that, as we age, the wear and tear on our bodies builds up. Our muscles gradually become less pliable. Our tendons (which attach our muscles to our bones) and our ligaments (which attach our bones to one another) become less able to rejuvenate and repair themselves. And then there are our bones themselves. Did you know that bone density begins to lessen as early as our late 30s? Both men's and women's bones become more porous with age, making them brittle and more likely to fracture. These are inevitable facts of our biological lives, and they account for some, but not all, of the reasons we lose flexibility as we age.

The main reason we lose flexibility as we get older is that we simply don't move enough. In fact, many of the functional losses associated with aging are not caused by the passage of time; they're actually the result of physical inactivity. The medical community has long had trouble distinguishing between the effects of aging and those of inactivity, but researchers are now learning that "being physically active makes your body on the inside more like a young person's."[9] A study published in 2011 found that "people don't have to lose muscle mass and function as they grow older. The changes that we've assumed were due to aging and therefore were unstoppable seem actually to be caused by inactivity. And that can be changed." The researchers added that they saw no reason why we can't reap the restorative benefits of exercise no matter our age when we start.[10]

What's at the heart of all this? Possibilities! Our bodies are ready and waiting for us to restore our flexibility in ways that are age appropriate, individually adaptable, and don't hurt. As we'll discover, yoga offers all these benefits and many more. It's an ideal way to increase our mobility and help assure that we can live active, independent lives for as long as providence allows.

CHAPTER 3

WHY CHOOSE YOGA FOR RESTORING FLEXIBILITY?

Yoga is a set of wellness practices that has its roots in ancient India. It can include breathing exercises, relaxation, and meditation, but we'll focus on *hatha*, or physical yoga, since that practice offers a direct pathway toward restoring flexibility. In hatha yoga, we mindfully move our bodies into and out of a variety of positions called postures or poses, and we experience beneficial stillness by holding these positions for a breath or two. In addition to being good for us, hatha yoga feels good because it's a journey through our comfort zone. We open and reach, but we don't force anything.

Because yoga is a low-impact form of exercise, it welcomes people of all ages, whether they're lifelong athletes or lifelong television enthusiasts. It's ideal for people with bone and joint conditions, and research is now showing that yoga also reduces the risk of cardiovascular disease. In fact, scientists have concluded that yoga is as good for our hearts as walking or bicycling. Unlike many forms of exercise, yoga also helps reduce stress and anxiety and, because no expensive equipment is needed, it can be practiced almost anywhere.[11]

Some people think of yoga as a form of stretching and, yes, it is that. But it's also much more. Traditional stretching usually targets one muscle or muscle group at a time, but yoga is holistic, uniting the body, the breath, and the mind. Even when we practice poses in which the primary benefit is greater flexibility, we're also reaping additional benefits, from muscle strengthening to breathing more efficiently.

Hatha yoga offers three specific types of health and fitness benefits: leading benefits that have a direct, positive impact on our physical fitness, enabling benefits that make it possible to reap the leading benefits, and well-being benefits that brighten our outlook on life, a key to healthy longevity. The three types are intertwined and inseparable, which is what makes yoga such a potent form of exercise.

THE LEADING BENEFITS OF YOGA

Though the following benefits are a foursome, one can follow from the other, and flexibility comes first. As you become more flexible, it's easier to become more agile—the two are kissin' cousins. If you're flexible and agile, it's easier to get stronger, and if you're flexible, agile, and strong, it's easier to reclaim the balance skills you had when you were younger. The leading benefits are:

- GREATER FLEXIBILITY. By gently lengthening our muscles and opening our joints, we increase our range of motion—how far we can stretch in any direction while remaining comfortable and pain-free. This increases our mobility and makes the movements of our daily lives safer and easier.

- ENHANCED AGILITY. Being agile means that we can change the direction and position of our bodies fluidly and without physical or mental strain. Because yoga includes bending, turning, rotating, and pivoting, it keeps us nimble.

- INCREASED STRENGTH. Yoga poses allow us to strengthen all our major muscles, which makes moving around easier. When our muscles are strong, we can move our joints with less effort, which makes us want to move more.

- IMPROVED BALANCE. As we age, our body's built-in balance systems may not work as well as they used to, but yoga offers easily learned techniques for reclaiming our balance skills. Good balance is essential to preventing falls as we age.

THE ENABLING BENEFITS OF YOGA

Not only do the following benefits make it possible for us to experience the poses and positions that form the heart of hatha yoga, they also enable us to lead healthier, fuller lives. The enabling benefits are:

- HEALTHIER POSTURE. Yoga helps us shed unhealthy postural habits that have built up over our lifetimes. Healthy posture helps ensure that we don't feel fatigued as quickly, we don't have as many aches and pains, and we can walk farther and longer.

- BETTER BREATHING. Yoga teaches us to keep our chests lifted and open, which helps us breathe more efficiently. Easy breathing exercises teach us to breathe more deeply and evenly, and the simple act of focusing on our breath relaxes us and reduces anxiety.

- ENHANCED MENTAL FOCUS. Yoga trains our body and mind to work better together, which is crucial to staying safe as we age. It also invites our complete attention, making it an ideal way to keep our minds sharp and active.

- IMPROVED ABILITY TO SENSE OUR BODIES IN SPACE. Our sense of proprioception (the ability of our nerves to perceive the location and orientation of our body parts as we move) can get a little rusty as we age, but yoga helps restore our ability to discern where our bodies are in space, a critical element in preventing falls.

THE WELL-BEING BENEFITS OF YOGA

Well-being—feeling content and satisfied with life—is strongly associated with healthy longevity, making the well-being benefits of yoga as important as the leading and enabling benefits. The well-being benefits are:

- CONNECTION TO OUR BODIES. Yoga invites us to reconnect with our physical selves. Too often we react to aging- or health-related changes in our bodies by disconnecting from our physicality, but yoga helps us regain confidence in our bodies as we age.

- STRESS REDUCTION. Because it teaches us to fully immerse ourselves in each present moment, yoga helps reduce stress and relieve anxiety. Both tend to arise when we dwell too much on past regrets or worry too much about the future.

- RELAXATION. By relaxing at the end of our yoga practice, we allow our bodies to absorb the benefits of our yoga poses so that we can resume our day feeling more alert and energetic. The ability to relax can actually reduce pain and improve the quality of our sleep as we age.[12]

CHAPTER 4

MAKING SURE THAT GENTLE YOGA IS SAFE FOR YOU

Before we begin, let's take a moment to make sure that gentle yoga-based exercise is safe for your unique body. When done in an age-appropriate, body-sensitive way that doesn't cause you pain, make you feel unsafe or insecure, or leave you breathless, the poses, practices, and techniques covered in this book are safe for most people. That's because they're gentle, sensible, and low impact. Even when bearing our weight, there's no jumping, running, or hopping. To benefit fully from some of them, you must be able to safely and comfortably lower yourself to the ground and get up again.

Osteoporosis and osteoarthritis are two common bone- and joint-related conditions that are usually diagnosed during or after midlife. Over 10 million American women and men have osteoporosis, putting them at greater risk of bone fractures, and over 27 million Americans have osteoarthritis, causing them at least some joint soreness and stiffness. The good news? Gentle yoga-based exercise is not only safe for people with either or both of these conditions, it's ideal for them. Yoga actually helps restore bone mass and, because it teaches us to bend and balance safely, it helps prevent fractures. Regular exercise has long been seen as an effective treatment for osteoarthritis, and research has shown that arthritis patients who exercise regularly have less discomfort in their joints than patients who do not.[13]

If you've had a shoulder, hip, or knee replacement, follow your doctor's or physical therapist's instructions for maintaining a safe range of motion at the replaced joint. If you're concerned about whether particular movements shown in this book are safe for your replaced joint, show *Restoring Flexibility* to your medical provider so that he or she can offer you informed, specific advice rather than generic recommendations.

The simple act of lowering to the ground and rising again does wonders for both our flexibility and agility, but be aware: Because we must resist gravity, rising is more difficult than lowering. Still, knowing how to safely get up after a fall could be a lifesaver. The two keys to coming down to the ground and getting up again safely and comfortably are moving gradually and mindfully (hurried, unthinking movements can lead to accidents) and maintaining a healthy, natural skeletal alignment while you're moving.

To learn how to safely lower yourself to the ground and rise again, turn to Appendix 1 (page 98) and follow the step-by-step instructions for "How to Safely Lower to the Ground and Get Up Again." If you're uncertain about whether you can rise again after lowering, follow the easy instructions for using a chair to help you.

If you still have questions, check with your doctor, physical therapist, or other healthcare professional to make sure that the yoga-based practices presented in *Restoring Flexibility* are safe for you.

CHAPTER 5

GETTING STARTED

In yoga, we stretch but we don't strain. By nature, we humans like to strive and reach, but in our modern world, where we no longer have to run like the dickens to avoid a hungry lion, our desire to strive can take us to unsafe extremes. To exercise safely, we must learn to listen to our bodies. Have no doubt—they'll tell us how far to go and when to stop. When we overstretch, our muscle fibers react by contracting and tightening, the exact opposite of the relaxed, open muscles we need in order to become more flexible.

There are three parts to every yoga pose: the movement into the pose, the stillness while holding the pose, and the movement out of the pose. Each is equally important, and in each you want to enjoy steadiness, alert comfort, and an even, natural breath. At the same time, you want to feel your joints and muscles responding, such as a gentle, healthy pull on the insides of your thighs when you widen your legs. A safe challenge may take you to the edge of your current range of motion—your comfort zone—but not beyond. It should feel good, and it should also feel like it's good for you. A challenge taken too far feels wrong—you can sense that it's not good for you.

GETTING BAREFOOT ON A STICKY MAT

Yoga is meant to be done barefoot on a sticky yoga mat so you can get traction while moving and holding still. Just as the treads of your car's tires need to hug the road, the soles of your feet need to hug the mat so that you don't hurt yourself as you try to keep from slipping. Your socks are smooth—they're made for slipping and sliding! Please don't do yoga in your socks! If you're squeamish about exposing your feet, remember that in the privacy of your own home, only you see your feet.

Yoga mats typically cost between $10 and $15 and are well worth the investment. Your mat will help keep you safe and comfortable, and you'll be much more satisfied with your yoga experience. Needless to say, if you own a mat, you'll be much more likely to use it!

SIX TIPS FOR A SAFE, ENJOYABLE PRACTICE

1: RESPECT YOUR BODY AS YOU PRACTICE. Your yoga poses are as individual as you are. There's no ideal or "correct" version of a yoga pose. There's only your healthiest, most comfortable, steadiest version.

2: MOVE GRADUALLY AND MINDFULLY. Focus your mind on each present moment. Try to avoid hurried, unthinking movements.

3: DON'T FORCE ANYTHING. Don't stretch beyond your individual range of motion. In yoga, it's not how far you go, it's *how* you go.

4: FINISH ONE POSE BEFORE STARTING THE NEXT. Yoga is not a race! Try to move naturally and fluidly, but do so at a pace that allows you to fully experience each pose. Yoga offers no benefit if all you're trying to do is get it over with.

5: HOLD A POSE ONLY AS LONG AS YOU FEEL COMFORTABLE AND STEADY IN IT. There's no ideal amount of time to be still in a yoga pose. One of the greatest joys of yoga is that you need not torture yourself for an assigned number of seconds, minutes, or repetitions.

6: THINK ABOUT HOW YOU FEEL IN EACH POSE. Are you comfortable? Do you feel a healthy response in your muscles and joints? Or do you feel anxious or tense? If so, ease up a little—you may have edged past your current comfort zone.

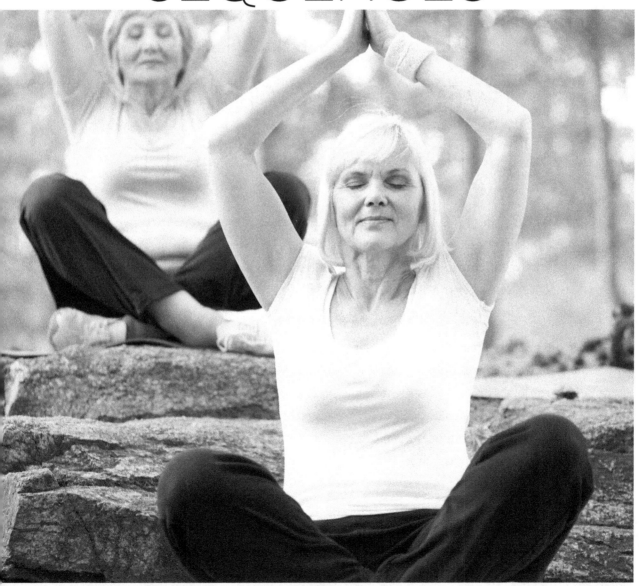

THE POSES
& PRACTICE
SEQUENCES

CHAPTER 6

LEARNING THE SEQUENCES: Two Approaches, Three Easy Steps

Yoga is easy. It's not difficult. The yoga flexibility poses presented in Part Two are specially designed and illustrated so that you can easily and safely learn them on your own. They're grouped into eight short, easy-to-learn sequences composed of several related poses meant to be practiced one after the other. Once you're familiar with the poses, each sequence should take between three and ten minutes.

The sequences are presented in the order in which they would be practiced in a well-rounded, head-to-toe yoga flexibility session. They begin with posture and breathing, continue with opening the joints and muscles in our upper body and spine, move through our mid-body with hip-opening sequences, maintain energy with a full-body agility sequence, and conclude with seated and reclining sequences meant to open the joints and muscles in our lower body. Each practice sequence is its own short book chapter so you can easily navigate among sequences.

WHERE TO START?
TWO APPROACHES

If you're not the kind of person who, upon seeing a swimming pool on a sunny summer day, jumps into the deep end without removing your street clothes, then you might appreciate having a couple sensible, practical ways to dive in to the process of restoring your flexibility using yoga-based exercise. One is sequence-based, where you focus on one group of related poses at a time, and the other is session-based, where you practice all the sequences in one of *Restoring Flexibility*'s suggested flexibility sessions.

SEQUENCE-BASED

If you want to become familiar with all eight practice sequences, thus assuring a head-to-toe flexibility program, try practicing the sequences in chapter order. This sequential approach allows you to be a learner in your own self-paced, personal yoga flexibility course. You can think of each sequence as one class, and you can move forward to the next class whenever you feel ready. Using this approach will fully prepare you for the Restoring Flexibility four-week program on page 84.

SESSION-BASED

If the sequential approach doesn't appeal to you, choose one of the flexibility sessions from the Restoring Flexibility four-week program on page 84 and practice it a few times to become familiar with its sequences and poses. Each session starts with a brief posture and breathing practice and continues with three additional practice sequences.

You can choose sessions that include sequences geared toward the least flexible areas of your body, sessions that are more or less vigorous depending on your energy level, or sessions that include exercises with which you're already familiar. If you're new to yoga, or have been away from it for a long time, just start with the four-week program's first session on page 87.

LEARNING THE SEQUENCES & POSES
IN THREE EASY STEPS

To learn a practice sequence and its component poses, try these three easy steps:

1: Review the numbered sequence that precedes the pose instructions so you can see the order in which the poses should be practiced.

2: Practice each pose, letting the bulleted instructions and illustrations guide you.

3: Practice the full sequence as slowly as you want, letting the at-a-glance numbered steps and thumbnail illustrations guide you.

Keep in mind that there's no wrong way and no one's going to criticize you. Whenever you've had enough, just move on to the next pose or sequence, or resume your practice tomorrow. Enjoy yourself. Don't rush, and don't force anything. The goal is not to master a particular pose or sequence, but to fully experience it. Yoga should feel like play, not like work.

Remember, every pose and sequence is designed to help restore your flexibility and increase your mobility.

CHAPTER 7

SEQUENCE 1:
Aligning Your Bones &
Centering Your Breath

We come into the world with perfect posture, and then life happens. Gradually, as we sit more and walk and run less, our habitual ways of standing and sitting become less natural. Yet, in order for our joints to function well, our bones need to be stacked in their most natural alignment. When standing, our ears should be over our shoulders, our shoulders should be over our hips, our hips should be over our knees, and our knees should be over our ankles. Our chin should be parallel to the ground as we look out at the world, not down at our feet. This keeps us stable and safe.

When our skeletons are misaligned, we use the wrong muscles in the wrong ways, which leads to fatigue, muscle weakness, joint stiffness, and loss of flexibility. Consider that 10-pound globe called your head. It's supported by the stack of 24 bones—the vertebrae—that comprise your spine. If you habitually carry your head in front of your shoulders rather than directly over them, you're forcing the small vertebrae in your neck to do a job that's actually meant for your entire spine. Not only must your neck and shoulder muscles work overtime but, as you age, it can become harder for you to hold your head upright.[14]

And that's not all. When you carry your head in front of your shoulders, your shoulders round forward, which causes your chest to compress. When your chest is compressed, you can't inhale as deeply or exhale completely. Many of us have gotten so used to a quicker, more shallow breath that we've forgotten what a really satisfying breath feels like. Did you know

that our brains associate quick, shallow breathing with fear and a long, slow breath with safety and security? Taking time to breathe well keeps us calm. We can also use our breath to help move our bodies, a valuable aide in restoring flexibility. When we let our breath do some of the work for us, our everyday movements, as well as our yoga poses, take less effort.

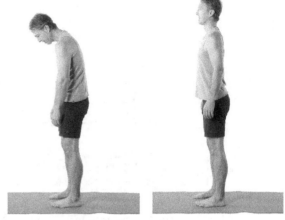

Unhealthy posture (left) and healthy posture (right)

Practice the following three-minute postural alignment and breath-centering sequence at the beginning of all your yoga flexibility sessions and you'll soon see that your posture is improving. (In fact, you may find yourself getting taller!) The sequence features Mountain Pose, the starting position for all the standing poses presented in this book. As you breathe in Mountain Pose and gently move with your breath, think about feeling alert without feeling tense or rigid.

THE SEQUENCE AT A GLANCE

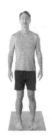

1. Ground and Grow into Mountain Pose

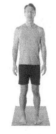

2. Breathe in Stillness

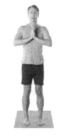

3. Move with Your Breath: Namaste Circles

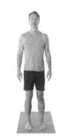

4. Return to Mountain Pose

HOW TO DO EACH POSE

MOUNTAIN POSE: GROUNDING

- Stand with your feet about hip-width apart. Look down and make sure the outsides of your feet are parallel to each other.

- Distribute your weight evenly over the bottoms of your feet—the outsides, the bottoms of your toes, the balls of your feet, and your heels.

- Stack your knees over your ankles.

- Bring the very tops of your thighs slightly back. Feel your lower belly lift slightly as you do this. This tiny movement will allow your hips to stack over your knees.

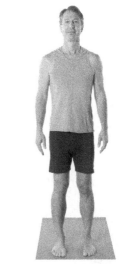

Mountain pose, front view

MOUNTAIN POSE: GROWING

- Grow taller by lengthening the sides of your body from your hips to your armpits.

- Gently lift your chest as you bring the top of your breastbone slightly back toward your spine. This tiny movement will allow your shoulders to draw back and stack above your hips.

- Stack your ears over your shoulders. Don't hang your head or snap your neck back.

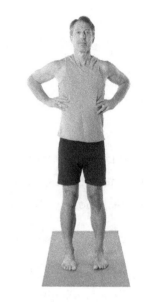

Lengthen sides of body.

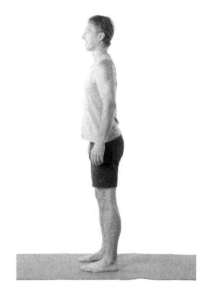

Mountain pose, side view

BREATHING IN STILLNESS

- Let your body settle into Mountain Pose.

- Close your eyes. Take five slow, long breaths.

- Open your eyes and take one slow, long breath.

- Close your eyes. Take five slow, long breaths.

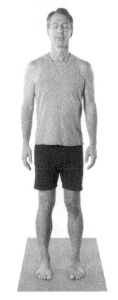

Breathe in stillness.

MOVING WITH YOUR BREATH: NAMASTE CIRCLES

- Inhale as you bring your arms straight out at shoulder level, palms facing up.

- Continue to inhale as your bring your arms up overhead, keeping them about shoulder-width apart.

- Touch your palms together overhead.

- Fully exhale as you lower your arms and touch your palms together at your breastbone. This position is called Namaste.

- You have now completed one full breath cycle. Lower your arms to your sides to return to Mountain pose and repeat two or three times.

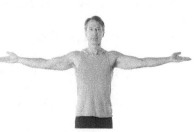

Inhale to bring arms out.

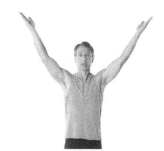

Continue inhaling to bring arms overhead.

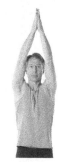

Touch palms together.

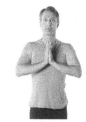

Exhale to Namaste.

ABOUT THE NAMASTE POSITION

Touching your palms together at your breastbone is called *namaste* in Sanskrit, the original language of yoga. It's used as a greeting or gesture of thanks in Buddhist cultures. Because Namaste invites us to rest our palms at the center of our chest—our center of gravity—it can help us feel balanced and grounded.

CHAPTER 8

SEQUENCE 2: Restoring Upper Body Flexibility

Here's a little something about our joints, those hundreds of places in our bodies where two bones come together. Each has a built-in range of motion—how far it can move in a particular direction—and a built-in method of movement. Some joints are designed to move from side to side, some backward and forward, some both ways, and some can rotate 360 degrees in a circle. To move our head forward and backward and to turn it to the left and right, we rely on the joints in the uppermost vertebrae of our spine, as well as the muscles that run alongside them. To move our arms through their circular range of motion, we rely on the ball-and-socket joints at our shoulders and the muscles that form our rotator cuff.

Given the sheer number of times we must move our head and arms in various ways throughout each day, we need our neck and shoulder joints to function as fully as possible. Yet it's these joints, along with the muscles that move them, that bear the brunt of the damage done by years of less-than-perfect posture. If you've ever had a stiff neck, you know what joint tightness and muscle fatigue feel like. In addition, most of us lose flexibility in our shoulder joints because we don't put our arms safely through their complete range of motion often enough. Thankfully, we can restore much of the flexibility we may have lost by intentionally sending these joints fully through their current range of motion. This should be done gently but frequently so that our range of motion gradually increases.

Take about seven minutes to practice the following five-position sequence designed to help restore your upper body flexibility. It starts with gentle stretching of your neck muscles and continues with arm circles designed to open your shoulder joints. Through slow, gentle movement, you'll also stretch both your upper chest and your upper back. Finally, you'll warm the muscles in your midsection through gentle side bends and safe twists.

THE SEQUENCE AT A GLANCE

Move fluidly, but hold each position long enough to fully experience it.

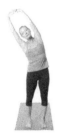 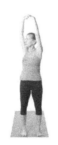 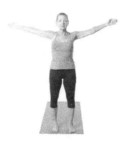 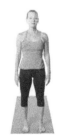

1. Mountain Pose

2. Gentle Neck Twist

3. Arm Circles

4. Bent-Elbow Chest and Back Stretch

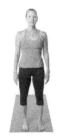 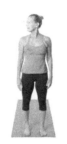 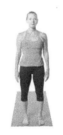 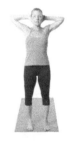

5. Standing Side Bend

6. Standing Twist

7. Return to Mountain Pose

8. Repeat the Sequence Once

HOW TO DO EACH POSE

GENTLE NECK TWIST

- Gently peek over your left shoulder. Take a breath.

- Return your head to center.

- Gently peek over your right shoulder. Take a breath.

- Repeat once.

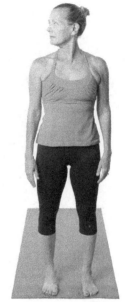

Gentle Neck Twist

ARM CIRCLES

- Bring your arms forward, up overhead, out to your sides, back, and down.

- Make three slow, continuous circles.

- Now, bring your arms back, out to your sides, up overhead, forward, and down.

- Make three slow, continuous circles.

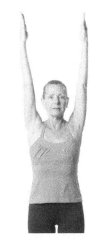

Arms up

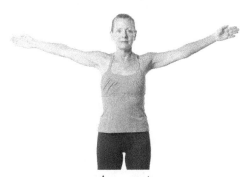

Arms out

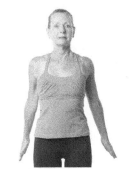

Arms back and down

BENT-ELBOW CHEST AND BACK STRETCH

- Raise your arms overhead and interlace your fingers, palms down.

- Now, rest your palms on the back of your head.

- Bring your elbows forward. Breathe.

- Bring your elbows back and out to your sides. Breathe.

- Repeat twice.

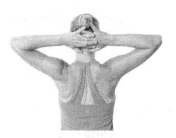

Palms on back of head

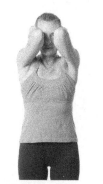

Elbows forward

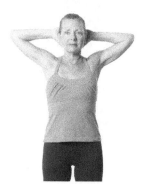

Elbows out and back

STANDING SIDE BEND

- Bring your arms overhead and interlace your fingers, palms down. Grow tall through the sides of your body and try to straighten your elbows as much as possible.

- Gently sway to the left.

- Return your arms to center.

- Gently sway to the right.

- Repeat once.

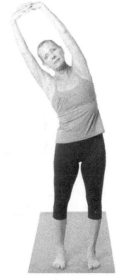

Standing Side Bend

STANDING TWIST

- Bring your arms overhead and interlace your fingers, palms down. Grow tall through the sides of your body and try to straighten your elbows as much as possible.

- Gently rotate your belly button a little to the left but not too far.

- Return to center.

- Gently rotate your belly button to the right.

- Return to center.

- Repeat once.

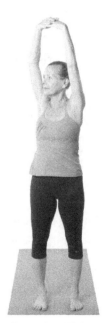

Standing Twist

CHAPTER 9

SEQUENCE 3: Restoring Spinal Flexibility

Exercise guru Joseph Pilates said that you're only as young as your spine is flexible, and his words ring as true today as they did in 1934, when he published his first fitness book. By moving our spine through its current range of motion, we allow the fluids stored in the cavities of our joints to wash over the discs that cushion the spaces between our vertebrae, keeping our spinal column flexible and mobile as we age.

All too often, back pain or stiffness that we assume must be caused by a sore muscle is actually caused by immobility in the joints of our spine. As we age, our discs become less absorbent, so they can easily become dehydrated. This lack of moisture can result in tight joints and loss of spinal mobility. The only way we can replenish the synovial fluids in our discs is through movement, so exercising our spine is essential to restoring flexibility.

The following seven-minute sequence invites you to flex and extend your entire spinal column. You'll open your vertebrae while moving with your breath, stretch the full length of your back by extending your arms and shoulders, and gently bend your back as you open the front of your body from your torso to your collarbone. Not only will these five gentle poses loosen your joints, they'll lengthen and relax the two sets of erector muscles that run up the length of your back alongside your spine, which will make it easier to fully and painlessly straighten your back after bending and reaching, two essential everyday movements.

This sequence offers a chance to lower to your hands and knees and get up again, which is immensely beneficial as long as you can do it safely. If you're uncertain about how to safely lower yourself to the ground and rise again, turn to Appendix 1 and follow the instructions for "How to Safely Lower to the Ground and Get Up Again."

THE SEQUENCE AT A GLANCE

Move fluidly, but hold each pose long enough to fully experience how it feels.

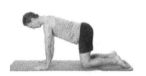

1. Tabletop Pose

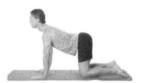

2. Cat/Cow Spinal Flexibility Flow

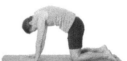

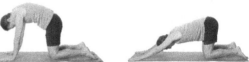

3. Extended Puppy Pose

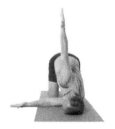

4. Threading the Needle with Optional Arm Raise, Left Arm Threaded

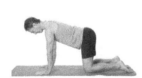

5. Return to Tabletop

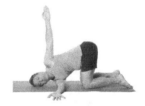

6. Threading the Needle with Optional Arm Raise, Right Arm Threaded

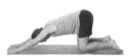

7. Repeat Extended Puppy Pose

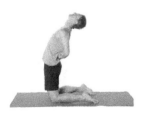

8. Camel Pose

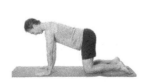

9. Return to Tabletop

HOW TO DO EACH POSE

TABLETOP

TIP: This pose will help strengthen your wrists. If your wrists get tired, put your fists, rather than your wrists, on the ground, as shown.

- On your hands and knees, stack your wrists under your shoulders.

- Stack your knees under your hips, keeping your ankles in line with your knees.

- Look down at the ground between your palms, keeping your ears in line with your shoulders. Don't hang your head or snap it back.

- Breathe naturally.

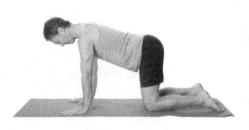

Tabletop, ears in line with shoulders

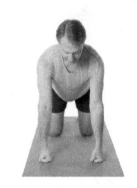

Tabletop, fists on ground

CAT/COW SPINAL FLEXIBILITY FLOW

- Inhale deeply as you lower your navel toward the ground, lift your chest, and look straight ahead. (Cow Pose)

- Now, exhale slowly as you press your belly button in toward your spine, arch your back, and look between your knees. (Cat Pose)

- Repeat twice for a total of three full breath cycles.

- From your third Cat Pose, inhale as you return to Tabletop.

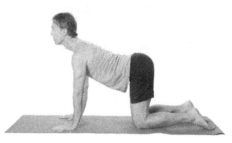

Inhale to Cow.

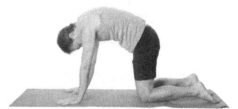

Exhale to Cat.

EXTENDED PUPPY

- Without moving your knees and hips, gently walk your palms forward, letting your shoulders and head naturally lower as you go.

- Be sure to keep your arms shoulder-width apart and your head in line with your arms.

- To stay within your comfort zone, choose a shorter or longer Extended Puppy.

- Take at least one full breath before walking your palms back to Tabletop.

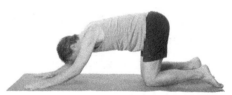

Shorter Extended Puppy

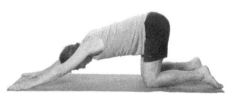

Longer Extended Puppy

THREADING THE NEEDLE
WITH OPTIONAL ARM OPENING

TIP: This pose is more comfortable if you take your glasses off before practicing it.

- From Tabletop, lower the back of your left forearm to the ground, palm up and fingers facing right.

- Slowly slide your left arm out to the right as you lower your left cheek to the mat. Let your cheek rest alongside your right palm. Take at least one full breath.

- Optional Arm Opening: Slowly reach your right arm straight up toward the ceiling. Take at least one full breath before lowering your arm.

- Slide your left arm back toward the left and return to Tabletop.

- Repeat, this time bringing your right forearm to the ground.

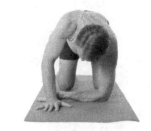

Lower forearm to mat.

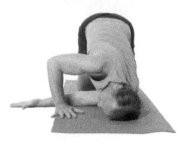

Needle is now threaded.

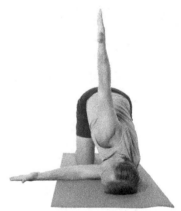

Optional arm opening

CAMEL

- From Tabletop, rise to stand on your knees.

- Rest your forearms comfortably on your back, as shown.

- Slowly and gently, stretch and lift the entire front of your body from the lowest part of your abdomen all the way to the top of your chest.

- Let your back gently bend as you lower your shoulders down toward the ground. Stay within your comfort zone, as shown.

- Keep your ears comfortably over your shoulders. Take at least one full breath.

- Return to Tabletop.

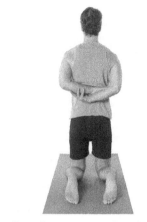

Rest forearms on back.

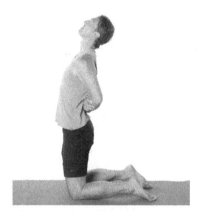

Camel with softer back bend

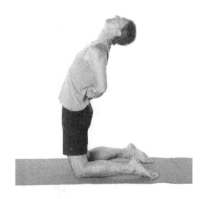

Camel with deeper backbend

CHAPTER 10

SEQUENCE 4: Restoring Hip Flexibility—Flexors

Healthy hip flexors—the muscles that enable us to bend forward—are critical in preserving mobility. They allow us to walk, bend our knees to sit down, straighten our knees to get up, lower our torso, arms, and shoulders closer to the ground, and fully rise again, all without aggravating our low back. Our two key sets of hip flexors are our psoas muscles, which begin at our mid-back and end just below our hip creases (the place where our legs meet our abdomen), and our hamstring muscles, which run down the backs of our thighs.

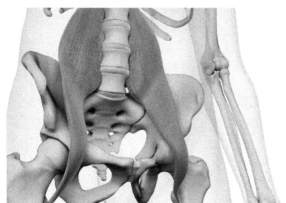

Psoas muscle

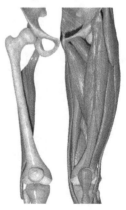

Hamstring muscles

Too much sitting over many years can eventually cause our psoas muscles to stay creased at our hips even after we rise, which can prevent us from rising to an upright position, eventually leading to the need for a walker. Too much sitting over many years can also cause our hamstrings to become tight and immobile. We tend to compensate for this by rounding from our waist when bending, which puts undue pressure on the muscles in our low back, causing discomfort, stiffness, and, all too often, chronic pain.

But remember, our bodies are resilient until we leave this life! These conditions are both preventable and more reversible than we might imagine. We can restore flexibility in our hip joints by gently but frequently coaxing our hip flexors to relax and open.

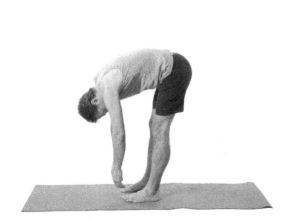
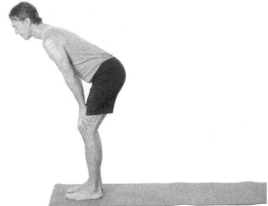

Unsafe, unhealthy way to bend forward   Safe, healthy way to bend forward

The three poses in this seven-minute sequence—the first of two sequences designed to help restore flexibility in our hips—invite us to stand with one leg extended behind our torso, which helps relax and lengthen our psoas muscles. The sequence's forward bends, called folds, allow us to safely relax and lengthen our hamstrings. By hinging (folding like an envelope flap) from our hip creases rather than rounding forward from our waist, we maintain the natural alignment and full length of our spine, which keeps our low back safe.

THE SEQUENCE AT A GLANCE

Move fluidly, but hold each pose long enough to fully experience how it feels.

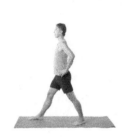

1. Extended Leg Stance, Left Leg Back

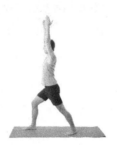

2. Warrior I, Right Knee Bent

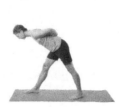

3. One-Sided Stretch with Forearms on Back, Left Leg Back

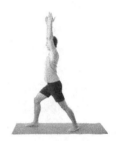

4. Repeat Warrior I, Right Knee Bent

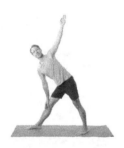

5. One-Sided Stretch with Twist and Arm Opening, Left Leg Back

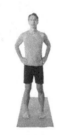

6. Mountain Pose

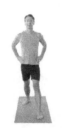

7. Extended Leg Stance, Right Leg Back

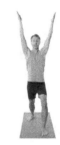

8. Warrior I, Left Knee Bent

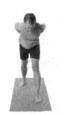

9. One-Sided Stretch with Forearms on Back, Right Leg Back

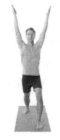

10. Repeat Warrior I, Left Knee Bent

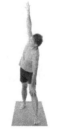

11. One-Sided Stretch with Twist and Arm Opening, Right Leg Back

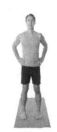

12. Mountain Pose

HOW TO DO EACH POSE

These instructions prompt you to bring your left leg back for each pose. The poses are done exactly the same way when you bring your right leg back.

EXTENDED LEG STANCE

- In Mountain Pose, place your hands on your waist.

- Keeping the outsides of your feet parallel to the edges of your mat, widen your feet slightly. They should be slightly wider than your hips.

- Step your left foot back behind your torso and lengthen your stance as much as is comfortable. Make sure that you feel balanced and stable.

- Turn your back foot out at about a 45-degree angle.

- Rotate your belly button to the right so your hips are even with each other and facing forward, like two headlights.

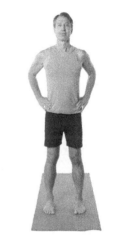

Hands on waist,
feet widened slightly

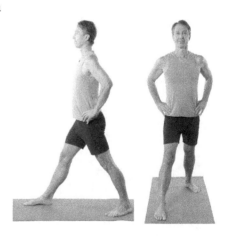

Extended Leg Stance,
side and front views

WARRIOR I

- From Extended Leg Stance, bend your right knee, stacking it over your right ankle.

- Make sure that your hips are still facing forward and your trunk is upright and tall, not bent forward.

- Raise your arms overhead. Your arms should be about shoulder-width apart.

- Take one or two full breaths as you find steadiness in the pose.

- Return your hands to your waist and straighten your right knee. You've now returned to Extended Leg Stance.

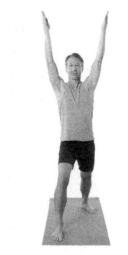

Warrior I, front view

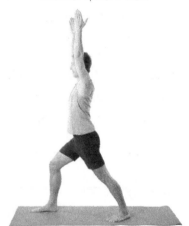

Warrior I, side view

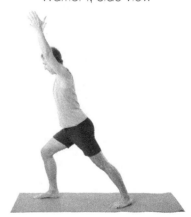

INCORRECT: Don't bend forward; keep trunk upright.

ONE-SIDED STRETCH

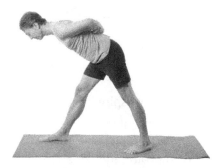

One-Sided Stretch

- In Extended Leg Stance, rest your forearms on your back, one on top of the other.

- Fold forward from your right hip crease. Keep your spine long and straight, folding only as deeply as is comfortable.

- Look down toward the ground, keeping your ears in line with your shoulders.

- Take one or two full breaths as you find steadiness in the pose.

- Rise and return your hands to your waist. You've now returned to Extended Leg Stance.

ONE-SIDED STRETCH WITH TWIST AND ARM OPENING

- From Extended Leg Stance, fold forward from your right hip crease, placing your palms on your right thigh.

- Keep your spine long and straight, folding only as deeply as is comfortable.

- Bring your left arm straight out at shoulder level.

- Rotate your belly button up and to the left as you extend your left arm up toward the ceiling.

- Take one or two full breaths as you find steadiness in the pose.

- To release the pose, return your left palm to your thigh, rise, and bring your hands to your waist.

- You have now returned to Extended Leg Stance.

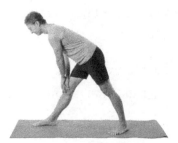

Fold forward and place palms on thigh.

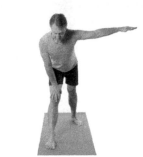

Bring left arm out at shoulder level.

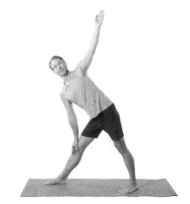

Rotate belly button and extend arm upward.

CHAPTER 11

SEQUENCE 5: Restoring Hip Flexibility—Rotators & Adductors

Have you ever wondered what kinesiology is? It's the study of human movement, and it can get enormously complicated, considering that each of us has 360 joints and 640 muscles! The sheer number of joints and muscles in our bodies not only indicates that we're designed to move in countless ways, it also indicates that many of these movements are complex, involving numerous joints and muscles at the same time.

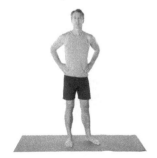
External hip rotation

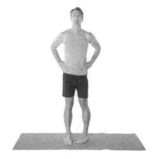
Internal hip rotation

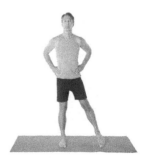
Hip adduction

Flexible hip joints are critical to physical mobility because they, along with our knee joints, make possible an array of complex movements that allow us to live independently and—though it probably goes without saying—stay safe as we move. In this seven-minute practice sequence, the second of two designed to help restore flexibility in our hip joints, we will focus on our rotators and adductors—the muscles that move the joints that allow us to widen our stance, rotate our legs inward toward the vertical middle of our body, and rotate them outward, away from our vertical middle.

Simply widening our legs enough to feel a healthy stretch along our inner thighs helps improve both balance and agility, two skills that are critical in preventing falls. Flexible muscles in our buttocks allow us to cross our legs comfortably and safely change direction as we move. Finally, we need relaxed, lengthened muscles on the outsides of our waists, hips, and thighs to protect our lower back while bending sideways. In fact, gentle side-bending may be a safe, comfortable alternative if you've been told to avoid bending forward because of a spinal condition or injury.

Two of the three poses in this wide-legged sequence invite you to turn one foot out at a 90-degree angle—an external rotation of your hip. To stay stable and balanced in this position, look at your feet, and make sure that the heel of your turned-out foot is aligned with the arch of your forward-facing, toes-slightly-turned-in foot. If you feel a little wobbly, your legs may be a little too far apart. Try a slightly narrower wide-leg stance that will still allow you to safely challenge yourself.

THE SEQUENCE AT A GLANCE

Move fluidly, but hold each pose long enough to fully experience how it feels.

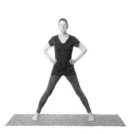

1. Wide-Leg Stance

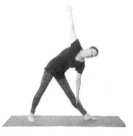

2. Triangle Pose, Left Foot Turned Out

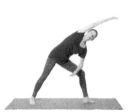

3. Side Angle Pose with Optional Arm Extension, Left Knee Bent

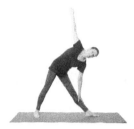

4. Repeat Triangle Pose, Left Foot Turned Out

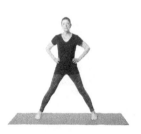

5. Return to Wide-Leg Stance

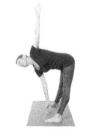

6. Wide-Leg Forward Fold with Twist and Left Arm Opening

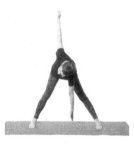

7. Wide-Leg Forward Fold with Twist and Right Arm Opening

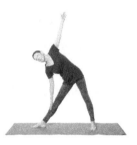

8. Triangle Pose, Right Leg Turned Out

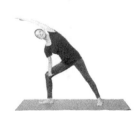

9. Side Angle Pose and Optional Arm Extension, Right Knee Bent

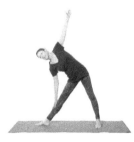

10. Repeat Triangle Pose, Right Leg Turned Out

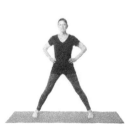

11. Return to Wide-Leg Stance

HOW TO DO EACH POSE

These instructions prompt you to turn your left foot out for Triangle and Side Angle. The poses are done exactly the same way when you turn your right foot out.

WIDE-LEG STANCE

- Begin in Mountain Pose, facing the long side of your mat.

- Place your hands on your waist, arms akimbo.

- Step your left leg out to the left and your right leg out to the right until you feel a healthy stretch along the insides of your thighs.

- Turn your toes in slightly. Your heels should be wider than your toes. This will enable you to bear your weight on the outsides of your feet and legs, which will keep you stable and balanced, just like an arch.

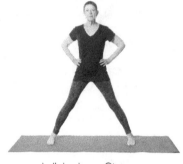

Wide-Leg Stance

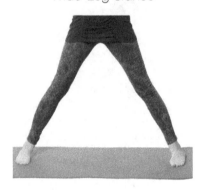

Turn toes in slightly.

TRIANGLE

- Bring your arms straight out to your sides at shoulder level, palms down.

- Turn your left foot out 90 degrees, aligning your left heel with your right arch.

- Shift your hips to the right and bend sideways to the left. Bend only as far as is comfortable.

- Gently rotate your belly button to the right and up so that your shoulders are even with each other. Don't round your right shoulder forward.

- Take one or two full breaths as you find steadiness in the pose.

- Gently rise, returning your hands to your waist.

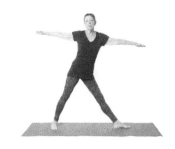

Turn left foot out 90 degrees and shift hips.

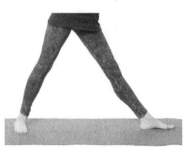

Align heel with arch.

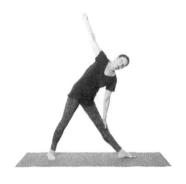

Softer Triangle

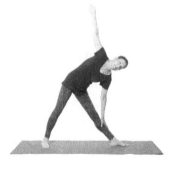

Deeper Triangle

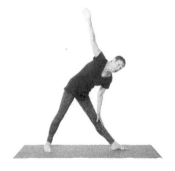

INCORRECT: Don't round shoulder forward.

SIDE ANGLE

- Make sure your left foot is turned out 90 degrees, your right toes are slightly turned in, and your hands are on your waist.

- Bend your left knee, stacking it over your left ankle. Make sure your knee is above your ankle, not to the left or right of it.

- Shift your hips to the right and bend sideways to the left. For a softer bend, rest your left palm on your thigh. For a deeper bend, rest your left forearm on your thigh, palm up.

- Gently rotate your belly button to the right and up so that your shoulders are even with each other. Don't bend your right shoulder forward.

- Take one or two full breaths as you find steadiness in the pose.

- Rise and straighten your left knee.

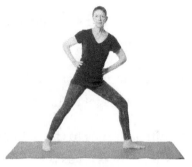

Bend knee.

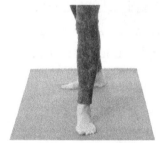

Stack knee over ankle.

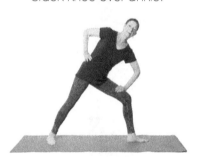

Softer Side Angle, palm on thigh

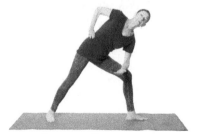

Deeper Side Angle, forearm on thigh

OPTIONAL ARM EXTENSION IN SIDE ANGLE

When practicing Side Angle, you can further lengthen the straight side of your body by extending your arm overhead. This is a deeper stretch, so explore it gently and remember that it's optional.

- In Side Angle, raise the inside of your right arm up past your face until it's alongside your right ear.

- Be sure to rotate your belly up and to the right so that your shoulders are even with each other, or as close to even as is comfortable.

- Take at least one full breath.

- Lower your right arm to your waist to return to Side Angle.

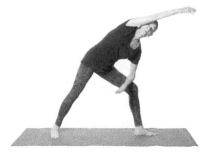

Raise your arm up past your face.

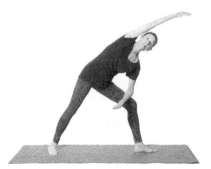

Side Angle with arm extension, arm alongside ear

WIDE-LEG FORWARD FOLD
WITH TWIST AND ARM OPENING

TIP: This pose invites you to bring the lowest part of your abdomen a little closer to the very tops of your thighs by folding from your hip creases.

- In Wide-Leg Stance, bring your arms straight out to your sides at shoulder level.

- Fold forward from your hip creases, keeping your arms out at shoulder level. Your back should be long and straight, not rounded.

- Gently rotate your belly button to the left and up, opening your left arm toward the ceiling.

- Take a breath as you experience the pose.

- Return to your forward fold, keeping your arms out at shoulder level.

- Repeat the twist and arm opening, this time rotating your belly button to the right and up.

- Rise and relax your arms.

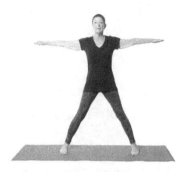

Arms out at shoulder level

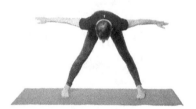

Fold forward halfway.

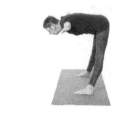

Keep a long, straight back.

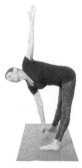

Rotate belly button up toward the ceiling.

CHAPTER 12

SEQUENCE 6: Restoring Agility— The Yoga Sun Salutation

The Sun Salutation is considered the most potent of all yoga sequences, and for good reason. It brilliantly unites five classic, whole-body poses to form a rhythmic flow that feels exhilarating and delivers the full flexibility benefits of all its component poses. And because it invites us to move fluidly from one position to the next, it powerfully enhances our agility—our capacity to easily and comfortably change the position of our body while remaining balanced, stable, and unafraid.

Preserving and restoring agility is one of the most effective ways to prevent falls as we age. If we're agile, it's not only easier to keep our balance, it's much easier to right ourselves if we accidentally move in a way that throws us off balance. How much agility is enough? We don't need the coordination of a basketball player or the balance skills of a gymnast. We only need to be agile enough to preserve our mobility and keep ourselves safe. If you're practicing the flexibility sequences in this book, you're already on the right track. There's a symbiotic relationship between flexibility and agility—when you become more flexible, it's much easier to become more agile.

There are countless adaptations of the yoga Sun Salutation, but we'll practice a gentle, age-respecting one that emphasizes both flexibility and agility. This Sun Salutation allows us to exercise our joints and muscles from head to toe, opening both the front and back of our body as we incrementally change body positions in order to journey down to the ground and back up again while keeping our hips in a stable, front-facing alignment. The order of the poses is no accident—each one easily follows the one that comes before it. The reason the Sun Salutation is such an effective way to improve agility is that it focuses as much on the movement from pose to pose as it does on the poses themselves.

You'll begin your journey by bringing your arms overhead and folding forward from your hip creases, just as we did in some of our earlier practices. You'll continue by bringing one and then both knees to the ground, ultimately lowering to your belly for a gentle backbend. To rise, you'll return to your knees and lift your hips for that classic yoga pose, Downward-Facing Dog. Finally, you'll return to a standing forward fold and slowly rise, once again bringing your arms overhead.

Sun Salutations are done in rounds because they include lunges. In the first half of the round, you'll bring your left leg back for your lunge and, in the second half, you'll bring your right leg back. When you've done the Sun Salutation sequence on each side, you've completed one full round. Once you're familiar with the poses, one round takes about seven minutes.

A quick tip: As you practice the Sun Salutation, stay within your current comfort zone and move from pose to pose slowly enough so that you can maintain an even, steady breath and comfortably change positions without straining or forcing anything.

THE SEQUENCE AT A GLANCE

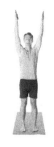

1. Upward Salute

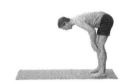

2. Forward Fold

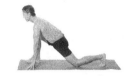

3. Low Lunge, Left Leg Back

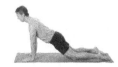

4. Low Plank

5. Lower to Belly

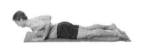

6. Low Cobra

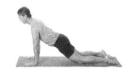

7. Rise to Low Plank

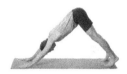

8. Downward-Facing Dog

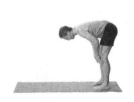

9. Rise to Forward Fold

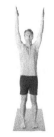

10. Rise to Upward Salute

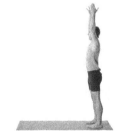

11. Repeat the entire sequence, this time bringing your right leg back for Low Lunge. You have now completed one full round.

HOW TO DO EACH POSE

UPWARD SALUTE

- Stand in Mountain Pose at the front of your mat.

- Bring your arms forward and up overhead, keeping them shoulder-width apart.

- Grow tall through the sides of your body and try to straighten your elbows as much as possible.

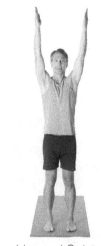

Upward Salute

FORWARD FOLD

- From Upward Salute, fold forward from your hip creases, bending your knees slightly. Fold only as deeply as is comfortable.

- As you fold, bring your arms forward and down. Let your hands rest on your knees.

- Keep your back long and flat. Don't round from your shoulders or waist.

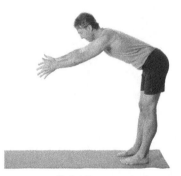

Fold Forward

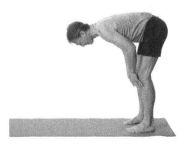

Rest hands on knees.

LOW LUNGE

These instructions prompt you to bring your left leg back. Low Lunge is done exactly the same way when you bring your right leg back.

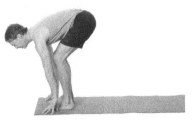

Bring fingertips to outsides of feet.

- From Forward Fold, bend your knees in a gentle squat and bring your fingertips to the outsides of your feet.

- Bring your left leg way back behind your left hand.

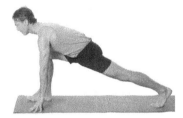

Bring leg back.

- Lower your left knee to the mat.

- Stack your right knee over your right ankle, as shown.

- Keep your hips facing forward and your ears in line with your shoulders. Don't hang your head or snap it back.

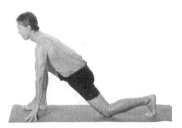

Lower back knee to mat.

- Breathe as you find steadiness in the pose.

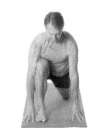

Stack front knee over front ankle.

LOW PLANK

- From Low Lunge, bring your right knee back so that it's even with your left knee.

- Make sure your shoulders are stacked over your wrists as shown, not back toward your knees.

- Press your belly button in toward your spine. Your belly should be firm, not hanging down toward the mat.

- Look down toward the mat, keeping your ears in line with your shoulders.

- Breathe as you find steadiness in the pose.

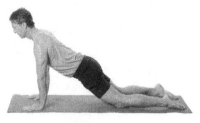

Stack shoulders above wrists and press belly button in toward spine.

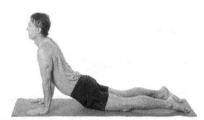

Don't let belly hang down toward mat.

LOWER TO BELLY

- From Low Plank, bend your elbows and gently lower your belly, chest, and chin to the mat.

- Keep your elbows close to your body. Try not to let them splay out.

- Keeping your elbows bent, let your fingertips rest alongside your chest.

- Take a resting breath.

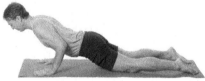

Bend elbows and gently lower to belly.

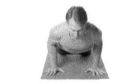

Keep elbows close to body.

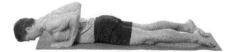

Rest fingertips alongside chest.

LOW COBRA

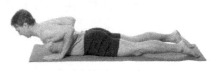

Low Cobra

TIP: You only need to lift your chest an inch or two off the mat for this very small backbend.

- Continue to rest your palms alongside your chest.

- Lift your chest slightly as you bring the bottoms of your shoulder blades in toward the front of your body. This gentle circular motion creates a small, soft bend in your upper back.

- Don't put any pressure on your palms. Let your chest and back do the work.

- Look down at the mat, keeping your ears in line with your shoulders as shown. Don't snap your head back.

- Take a breath.

- Gently lower your chest and head back to the mat.

DOWNWARD-FACING DOG

- From your belly, rise to Low Plank.

- Turn your toes under and lift your knees and hips up off the mat.

- Press into the mat with the heels of your hands as you bring your shoulders back and lengthen your arms. Stretch only as deeply as is comfortable.

- Straighten your legs or keep your knees slightly bent, whichever is more comfortable.

- Rest your head between your elbows, keeping your ears in line with your arms. Don't hang your head.

- Take at least one full breath.

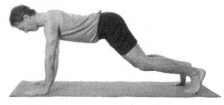

Lift knees and hips off mat.

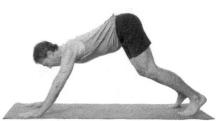

Bring shoulders back and lengthen arms.

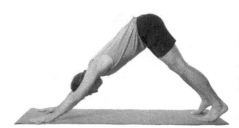

Downward-Facing Dog, legs straight

RISE TO FORWARD FOLD

- From Downward-Facing Dog, bend your knees and walk your feet forward a step or two.

- Keeping your knees bent, walk your hands toward your feet a step or two.

- Lift your fingertips up off the mat and rest your hands on your knees, keeping your knees slightly bent.

- You have now returned to Forward Fold.

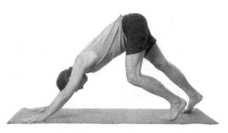

Walk feet toward hands.

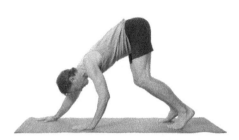

Walk hands toward feet.

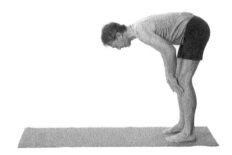

Return to Forward Fold.

RISE TO UPWARD SALUTE

- From Forward Fold, slowly rise to standing, bringing your arms forward and all the way up overhead to return to Upward Salute.

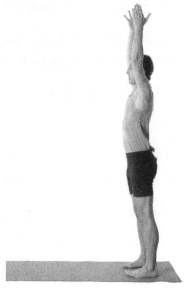

Rise, bringing arms overhead.

CHAPTER 13

SEQUENCE 7:
Restoring Lower
Body Flexibility

When we think of restoring lower body flexibility, we might think first of our hip joints, as we've explored in our previous practices. We might also be aware of tightness or fatigue in our thigh muscles or knees when we climb steps, or we might feel strained in our mid-body when we bend and twist to reach for something above or below us. Everyday life doesn't offer many chances to stretch our calf muscles and yet, if you've ever had a cramp in your calf, you know how painful it can be. Yoga can be a real benefit when it comes to restoring flexibility in our waists, thighs, knees, and calves.

Then there are our feet, those two steadfast structures that spend most of their waking hours trapped in our shoes. They long to be free! We give far too little attention to keeping our ankles, feet, and toes flexible and strong, especially as we age. If you've ever had a painful pull in the back of your ankle—your Achilles tendon—you know only too well where the expression "Achilles heel" comes from. And how about those nasty toe cramps! Including our ankles, feet, and toes in a yoga flexibility practice carries significant health benefits, from improved circulation to better balance to fewer foot cramps and ankle strains.

This lower body flexibility practice features some movements and positions from our standing practices, but because they're done in a seated position, they can feel restful and restorative. How does a more soothing flexibility practice benefit us? First, it situates us on the ground so that we don't need to bear our weight or resist gravity as we practice. Second, because seated poses require less muscle energy, we can find ease and comfort for a longer time, which allows us to stretch more deeply while staying safe.

This six-minute sequence focuses on gentle forward folds, side bends, and hip-opening poses, including Bound Angle, a classic yoga posture in which we widen our knees in order to bring the soles of our feet as close to each other as is comfortable. This pose is meant to gradually open your groin muscles, so you'll feel a gentle pull along the insides of your thighs while practicing it. Be mindful of how your thighs feel, and release your Bound Angle when that gentle pull begins to feel like too much.

You may practice the optional flexibility exercises for your ankles, feet, and toes at the beginning or end of the sequence, or at both times.

THE SEQUENCE AT A GLANCE

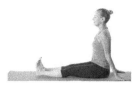

1. Staff Pose

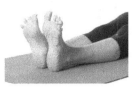

2. Optional: Exercise Ankles, Feet, Toes (page 74)

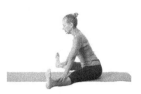

3. Seated Wide-Leg Forward Fold

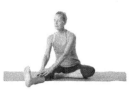

4. Head Toward Knee, Left Knee Bent

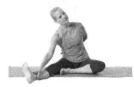

5. Revolved Head Toward Knee, Left Knee Bent

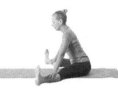

6. Repeat Seated Wide-Leg Forward Fold

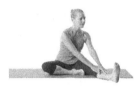

7. Head Toward Knee, Right Knee Bent

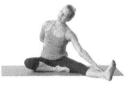

8. Revolved Head Toward Knee, Right Knee Bent

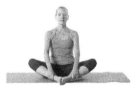

9. Bound Angle Pose

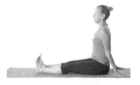

10. Return to Staff Pose

HOW TO DO EACH POSE

These instructions prompt you to bend your left knee for Head Toward Knee and Revolved Head Toward Knee. The poses are done exactly the same way when you bend your right knee.

STAFF POSE

TIP: Your "sitting" bones are located at the lowest part of your buttocks, just above the backs of your thighs.

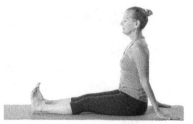

Staff Pose using palms
for support

- Sit on your "sitting" bones with your legs straight out in front of you and your toes pointed upward. Don't sit on your tailbone.

- Grow tall through your torso by lengthening the sides of your body from your hips to your armpits.

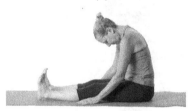

INCORRECT: Unhealthy
seated posture

- Gently lift your chest as you bring the top of your breastbone slightly back toward your spine.

- Stack your ears over your shoulders.

- To avoid rounding your shoulders, walk your hands two or three inches behind your shoulders and use your palms for support, as shown.

SEATED WIDE-LEG FORWARD FOLD

TIP: This pose is a gentle movement in which you lean forward in order to bring the very bottom of your abdomen a little closer to the very tops of your thighs.

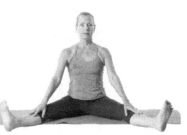

Keep toes in line with knees and pointing upward.

- From Staff Pose, widen your legs as much as is comfortable. Keep your toes in line with your knees and point them upward.

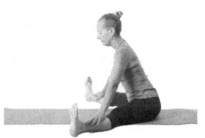

- Fold forward from your hip creases as you gently slide your palms down your thighs.

- Keep your shoulders in line with your hips. Don't round your shoulders forward. Don't hang your head.

- Take two or three full breaths as you relax in the pose.

Gently fold forward.

HEAD TOWARD KNEE

- From your wide-legged seated position, bend your left knee and place the sole of your left foot near the inside of your right thigh.

- Rotate your belly button to the right so that you're looking out over your right (straight) leg.

- Fold forward from your right hip crease as you gently slide your palms down your right leg.

- Keep your shoulders in line with your hips. Don't round your shoulders forward. Don't hang your head.

- Take two or three full breaths as you relax in the pose.

- Release your forward fold, but keep your left knee bent so that you're in position for Revolved Head Toward Knee.

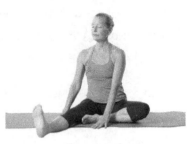

Place sole of foot near inside of opposite thigh.

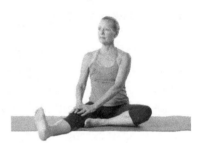

Rotate belly button and look out over straight leg.

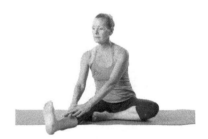

Gently fold forward.

REVOLVED HEAD TOWARD KNEE

- With your left knee bent, rotate your belly button to the left so that you're looking out over your left (bent-knee) leg.

- Rest your left forearm on your back.

- Gently bend sideways to the right, sliding your palm down your right (straight) leg as you go. Bend only as deeply as is comfortable.

- Make sure that your shoulders are in line with each other. Don't round your left shoulder forward.

- Take two or three full breaths as you relax in the pose.

- Release your side fold and return to Staff Pose.

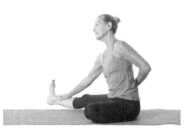

Rotate belly button and look out over bent knee. Rest left forearm on back.

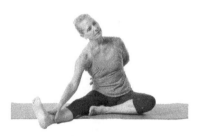

Bend sideways over straight leg.

BOUND ANGLE

- From Staff Pose, bend your knees and bring the soles of your feet as close to each other as is comfortable.

- See if you can comfortably touch one sole to the other. If that's not comfortable, let your soles rest facing each other, as shown.

- Keep your trunk upright and sit on your sitting bones, not on your tailbone.

- Rest your hands on your knees as you look forward. Keep your ears stacked over your shoulders.

- Take at least two or three breaths as you relax in the pose.

- Return to Staff Pose.

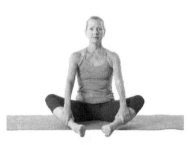

Bring soles of feet closer to each other.

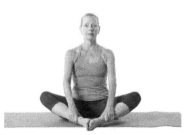

If comfortable, touch soles of feet to each other.

HOW TO DO THE ANKLES, FEET, &
TOES EXERCISES

ANKLES, FEET, & TOES FLEXIBILITY SEQUENCE

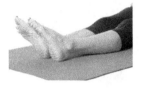

1. Rotate your ankles three times clockwise and three times counter-clockwise.

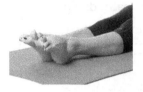

2. Wiggle your toes.

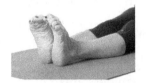

3. Curl your toes.

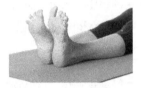

4. Spread your toes.

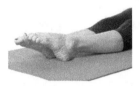

5. Point toes strongly away from ankles.

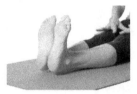

6. Point toes strongly toward ankles. You should feel a stretch in your calf muscles.

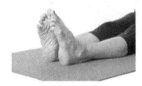

7. Bring soles of feet closer to each other.

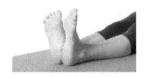

8. Move soles of feet farther away from each other.

CHAPTER 14

SEQUENCE 8:
Reclining Joint Releases
& Muscle Relaxation

Did you know that in yoga, every body position is ideal for restoring flexibility? So, though it may seem counterintuitive, we can significantly increase our flexibility even when we're relaxing on our back. How is this possible? When we're reclining, we're no longer defying gravity, so we don't have to worry about our posture or balance. We can safely bend and stretch in ways that may be beyond our anatomical limits when standing or sitting. Lying on our back not only allows us to release and relax different joints and muscles, it also allows us to comfortably—even effortlessly—hold poses that might be painful or contraindicated if done seated or standing, whether because of immobility in a joint, muscle weakness, balance issues, or an injury.

During reclining sequences, we can take advantage of "passive" stretching, in which we allow our joints and muscles to naturally open and release simply by lying still in a comfortable position and letting the force of gravity act on us. Not surprisingly, poses that we previously practiced standing or sitting affect our bodies differently when done on the back. Most feel more restful, but as you'll discover, some retain a pleasant, comfortable level of energy. This is why reclining yoga poses are as important to restoring flexibility as standing and seated poses.

Our reclining sequence opens and closes with a full-body stretch that—no kidding!—will feel as good to you as it does to your favorite cat. In between, you'll enjoy a bent-knee twist that invites you to lengthen the pectoral muscles in your chest, you'll bring your knees closer to your chest so that you can relax the muscles in your low back, and you'll reprise the groin-opening Bound Angle Pose, this time lying down.

Because they calm us down, reclining sequences are often done at the end of a yoga session and are usually followed by a few minutes of relaxation. Simply relaxing on your back with your eyes closed, even for two or three minutes, helps your muscles and joints "remember" the benefits of your flexibility practices. The classic yoga relaxation posture, called Savasana, is included in this sequence. As long as your low back, neck, and head are supported and comfortable, Savasana requires virtually no muscle effort, which is why it's so refreshing. When lying in Savasana, you may want to use a pillow or folded towel to support your neck and head.

A quick tip: You don't need to wait until the end of your flexibility session to practice this soothing sequence. It can be done anytime: as an alternative to an afternoon nap, as a relaxing exercise series in the evening before bed, and even as a gentle morning wake-up routine that you can do while you're in bed.

THE SEQUENCE AT A GLANCE

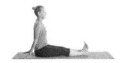

1. Begin in Staff Pose

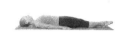

2. Lower to Back

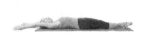

3. Full-Body Stretch (twice)

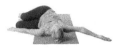

4. Reclining Bent-Knee Twist with Arm Extension, Knees Facing Left

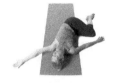

5. Reclining Bent-Knee Twist with Arm Extension, Knees Facing Right

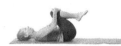

6. Knees Toward Chest (twice)

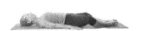

7. Reclining Bound Angle

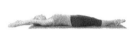

8. Full-Body Stretch (twice)

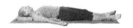

9. Savasana

HOW TO DO EACH POSE

All poses are done while lying on your back.

LOWERING TO YOUR BACK

- Begin in Staff Pose.

- Ease back and down to your forearms, as shown.

- Gently lower your head to the mat.

- Rest your arms alongside your body.

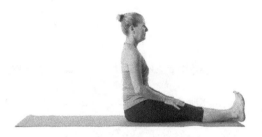

Begin in Staff Pose.

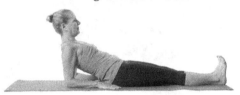

Ease down to forearms.

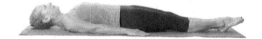

Lower head to mat.

FULL-BODY STRETCH

- Inhale, bringing your arms straight up overhead and pointing your toes away from your body.

- Make your inhalation long and slow so that you can fully stretch your entire body.

- Exhale slowly, bringing your arms to rest alongside your body and relaxing your feet.

- Repeat once.

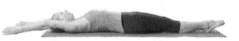

Bring arms overhead and point toes away from body.

RECLINING BENT-KNEE TWIST WITH ARM EXTENSION

- Keeping your legs close together, bend your knees and lift your feet off the mat.

- Slowly roll to your left, letting your right hip come off the ground. Let your legs gently fall toward the ground. Don't resist gravity.

- Gently lower your right shoulder closer to the mat.

- Slide your right arm along the ground, palm up, bringing it out and up toward your head. Slide only as far as is comfortable.

- Take at least three full breaths as you relax in the pose.

- Lift your knees, bringing them back to center. Repeat, this time rolling to your right.

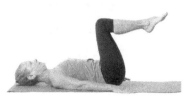

Bend knees and lift feet off mat.

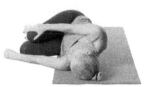

Roll to left.

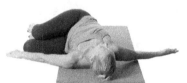

Lower right shoulder closer to mat.

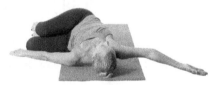

Slide right arm out and up.

KNEES TOWARD CHEST

TIP: To massage different areas of your low back and buttocks, try bringing your knees closer to and farther away from your chest and rolling from side to side in the pose.

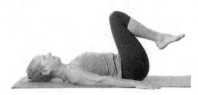

Bring knees closer to chest.

- Bend your knees.

- Slowly bring them closer to your chest.

- If it feels comfortable, place your hands on the front of your knees and use your arms to gently pull your knees closer to your chest.

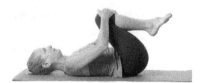

Use arms to pull knees closer to chest, if comfortable.

- Take at least three full breaths as you relax in the pose.

- Relax your knees back down to the mat.

- Repeat once.

RECLINING BOUND ANGLE

- Widen your knees and bring the soles of your feet as close to each other as possible.

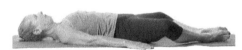

Reclining Bound Angle, soles of feet facing each other

- See if you can comfortably touch one sole to the other. If that's not comfortable, let your soles rest facing each other, as shown.

- Let gravity help you relax your knees down toward the mat. Your knees will probably not touch the ground.

- Take at least three breaths as you relax in the pose.

- You'll feel a good stretch through your inner thighs and groin area, so remain in the pose only as long as you feel comfortable.

SAVASANA

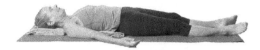

Savasana

- Make yourself comfortable. If you want, put a pillow or folded towel under your neck and head for support.

- Let your legs gently splay apart.

- Widen your arms far enough away from your trunk so that you feel comfortable with your palms facing up.

- Close your eyes and breathe naturally, letting your entire body relax.

- Let your mind clear out. See if you can stay in the present moment. If your mind wanders, just guide it to pleasant, relaxing places.

- Relax in Savasana for at least two or three minutes, or as long as you wish.

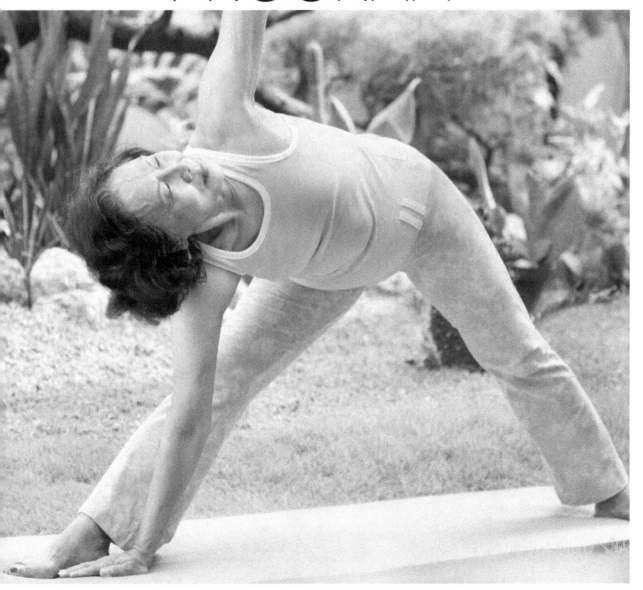

PART THREE

THE RESTORING FLEXIBILITY PROGRAM

CHAPTER 15

THE RESTORING FLEXIBILITY FOUR-WEEK PROGRAM

Restoring our flexibility is a process—it happens gradually over time. The four-week program is a tool specifically designed to support this process. It allows you to expand your comfort zone progressively, session by session and week by week. Each session builds on poses and sequences you practiced in previous sessions, so even when you're practicing new poses, you'll be in familiar territory.

Each of the eight suggested yoga flexibility sessions is composed of four practice sequences, and each is designed to take 20 to 25 minutes. While you're learning the poses and sequences, they may take a little longer, but after you practice a sequence three or four times, you'll be pleasantly surprised at how well you remember the poses.

Each session begins with Sequence 1: Aligning Your Bones and Centering Your Breath, and continues with three additional sequences that vary from session to session. Don't shortchange Sequence 1—it will make the other three sequences in your session easier. Taking a moment to practice healthy posture and breathing not only sets the stage for a safe, enjoyable flexibility session, it greatly improves our health off the mat.

Not only do the eight practice sequences in the program vary according to the areas of our body on which they focus, they also vary according to how much physical and mental exertion they require. To guide you, each sequence has an "activity level" rating—either 1, 2, or 3:

1. Relaxed, featuring greater stillness, very gentle movements, or less resistance to gravity.

2. Comfortably active, featuring standing or kneeling poses that easily flow from one pose to the next without moving your base of support.

3. Active and agile, featuring the Sun Salutation, in which the movement from one position to the next is as important to the sequence as the poses themselves.

Activity level ratings are included for each sequence in each of the flexibility sessions.

THE RESTORING FLEXIBILITY TOOL KIT

The following tools are designed to make it easy for you to begin, continue, and—yes!—progress beyond your four-week yoga flexibility program.

- **Eight 21-Minute, 22-Minute, and 23-Minute Flexibility Sessions**

  These are the components of the four-week Restoring Flexibility program. They're listed on the Four-Week Yoga Flexibility Program at a Glance on page 87. You can follow the program progressively, as suggested, or pick and choose sessions to create your own program.

- **Four 9-Minute, 10-Minute, and 12-Minute Mini Flexibility Sessions**

  These include a Morning Mini, a Midday Mini, an Evening Mini, and a Go-Anywhere Mini that you can easily do when you're away from home. They're listed in the Mini Sessions at a Glance on page 88. You can add any of these to your program or substitute one of them for a longer session.

- **Four-Week Program at a Glance**

  This handy one-page reference chart on page 87 shows the eight suggested sessions in the order in which the progressive four-week program should be followed. Each session's listing includes the name of each practice sequence, the number of minutes each sequence might take once you're familiar with the component poses, and each sequence's activity level rating—1, 2, or 3.

- **Mini Sessions at a Glance**

  This handy one-page reference chart on page 88 shows the four mini-sessions—morning, midday, evening, and go-anywhere. It includes the same at-a-glance information as the regular sessions.

- **Eight Session Guides**

  Appendix 2 (page 105) features eight session guides. Each guide shows the numbered steps for all four practice sequences in that session, exactly as shown in each sequence's chapter in this book. Keep your guide handy as you practice. It will help you remember each sequence's component poses so that you won't need to keep referring back to each individual chapter in this book.

- **Four Session Guides for the Mini Sessions**

  Appendix 2 also contains session guides for the mini sessions that start on page 122. Each one-page guide shows the same information as the guides for the regular sessions.

THE RESTORING FLEXIBILITY
FOUR-WEEK PROGRAM AT A GLANCE

SESSION 1: WEEK 1, DAY 1

SEQUENCE	MINUTES	ACTIVITY LEVEL
Aligning/Centering, p. 23	3	1
Upper Body, p. 30	6	1
Lower Body, p. 67	6	1
Reclining/Relaxing, p. 75	6	1
SESSION TOTALS	**21**	**4**

SESSION 2: WEEK 1, DAY 2

SEQUENCE	MINUTES	ACTIVITY LEVEL
Aligning/Centering, p. 23	3	1
Upper Body, p. 30	6	1
Hips: Flexors, p. 42	7	2
Lower Body, p. 67	6	1
SESSION TOTALS	**22**	**5**

SESSION 3: WEEK 2, DAY 1

SEQUENCE	MINUTES	ACTIVITY LEVEL
Aligning/Centering, p. 23	3	1
Spine, p. 36	7	2
Hips: Rotators, p. 49	7	2
Reclining/Relaxing, p. 75	6	1
SESSION TOTALS	**23**	**6**

SESSION 4: WEEK 2, DAY 2

SEQUENCE	MINUTES	ACTIVITY LEVEL
Aligning/Centering, p. 23	3	1
Spine, p. 36	7	2
Hips: Flexors, p. 42	7	2
Lower Body, p. 67	6	1
SESSION TOTALS	**23**	**6**

SESSION 5: WEEK 3, DAY 1

SEQUENCE	MINUTES	ACTIVITY LEVEL
Aligning/Centering, p. 23	3	1
Upper Body, p. 30	6	1
Sun Salutation, p. 57	7	3
Reclining/Relaxing, p. 75	6	1
SESSION TOTALS	**22**	**6**

SESSION 6: WEEK 3, DAY 2

SEQUENCE	MINUTES	ACTIVITY LEVEL
Aligning/Centering, p. 23	3	1
Hips: Rotators, p. 49	7	2
Lower Body, p. 67	6	1
Reclining/Relaxing, p. 75	6	1
SESSION TOTALS	**22**	**5**

SESSION 7: WEEK 4, DAY 1

SEQUENCE	MINUTES	ACTIVITY LEVEL
Aligning/Centering, p. 23	3	1
Spine, p. 36	7	2
Sun Salutation, p. 57	7	3
Reclining/Relaxing, p. 75	6	1
SESSION TOTALS	**23**	**7**

SESSION 8: WEEK 4, DAY 2

SEQUENCE	MINUTES	ACTIVITY LEVEL
Aligning/Centering, p. 23	3	1
Upper Body, p. 30	6	1
Hips: Rotators, p. 49	7	2
Lower Body, p. 67	6	1
SESSION TOTALS	**22**	**5**

MINI SESSIONS AT A GLANCE

MORNING MINI

SEQUENCE	MINUTES	ACTIVITY LEVEL
Lower Body, p. 67	6	1
Upper Body, p. 30	6	1
SESSION TOTALS	**12**	**2**

MIDDAY MINI

SEQUENCE	MINUTES	ACTIVITY LEVEL
Aligning/Centering, p. 23	3	1
Sun Salutation, p. 57	7	3
SESSION TOTALS	**10**	**4**

EVENING MINI

SEQUENCE	MINUTES	ACTIVITY LEVEL
Lower Body, p. 67	6	1
Reclining/Relaxing, p. 75	6	1
SESSION TOTALS	**12**	**2**

GO-ANYWHERE MINI

SEQUENCE	MINUTES	ACTIVITY LEVEL
Aligning/Centering, p. 23	3	1
Upper Body, p. 30	6	1
SESSION TOTALS	**9**	**2**

CHAPTER 16

BUILDING THE PROGRAM INTO YOUR LIFE

You'll benefit most from your yoga flexibility program if you practice regularly and frequently—in other words, if you integrate your practice into your everyday life. For most of us, though, that's easier said than done, especially if we're not used to regular exercise. When it comes to restoring and maintaining flexibility, you can't substitute intensity (practicing harder) or duration (practicing longer) for frequent, regularly scheduled practice sessions that don't end after completing a four-week program, but instead become an integral part of your healthiest, happiest life. And please remember—a regular, ongoing exercise habit is important at all ages, but it is critical after midlife.

A sustainable yoga flexibility program should meet three essential criteria:

1. It should be enjoyable. It shouldn't be boring or tedious. It should be a part of your day to which you can look forward. It should make you feel like you're doing something good for yourself, both during and after each practice session. It shouldn't deplete your energy, and it should leave you feeling better, not worse, than when you started.

2. It should feel right for your body. It should never hurt. It should offer both the degree of challenge (intensity) and the types of challenges (movements, poses, and positions)

that your body can welcome and accept. It should offer an appropriate level of physical and mental exertion, depending on variables like time of day and how you're feeling that day.

3. It should fit comfortably into your schedule. The sessions have to be short enough—20 minutes or so is fine—so that you won't feel tempted to skip your practice. If you make a promise to yourself to exercise twice a week, schedule your flexibility sessions on days and at times when you're most likely to keep that promise.

FITTING YOUR FLEXIBILITY PRACTICE INTO YOUR SCHEDULE

Integrating a new habit, no matter how positive or enjoyable, into our daily lives is a challenge at any stage of life, whether we have a sometimes-too-busy schedule or a daily routine that we're used to and with which we've become comfortable and contented. As you think about when you want to schedule your twice-weekly flexibility sessions, consider starting with these tried-and-true strategies for creating and sustaining any positive lifestyle habit:

1. Replace a habit you want to shed with your yoga flexibility habit. For example, think of how much television you watch and when you watch it. Remember, adding a new habit to those we already have can make us feel busier, and we can come to resent the new habit.

2. Give your yoga flexibility practice the same priority as you would a doctor's appointment and treat it as a prescription. An increasing number of doctors actually do prescribe gentle yoga-based exercise to patients who can no longer escape the fact that they must get moving.

3. Enlist a friendly nag. Tell someone you trust that you're going to start practicing yoga-based exercise and invite them to be your "friendly nag"—the person who can give you a good-natured poke if you feel yourself falling away from your flexibility practice.

TIPS FOR CREATING A SUSTAINABLE PRACTICE SCHEDULE

- Try to schedule your twice-weekly flexibility sessions at the same time of day and on the same days of the week, whether that's Tuesdays and Thursdays at 9:30 a.m., Saturdays and Tuesdays at 4:30 p.m., or whatever combination works for you. If it isn't possible to schedule both your sessions at the same time of day because of your work schedule, grandchild care responsibilities, or other hard-wired commitment, try practicing one weekend morning and one weekday late afternoon or evening.

- Yoga wisdom—and common sense—hold that full-bodied, energetic poses and practices are well suited to daytime, when your energy reserves are at their highest, and calming poses and practices (those that don't require your body to resist gravity as much) are well suited to the evening hours. Look at the total activity-level rating for each session—that's the sum of the activity-level ratings for each of the sequences in the session—to see if you can schedule your program's more-active sessions for mornings or early afternoons and its less-active sessions for late afternoons or evenings.

- Be as kind to yourself as possible. Don't try to practice at times when getting up and moving is harder—for instance, shortly after a meal, when you feel the urge for an afternoon catnap, or during your favorite television show.

- No matter what time of day or evening you practice, try to do so on an empty or almost-empty stomach—at least an hour after a meal.

CHAPTER 17

ADAPTING THE PROGRAM TO MEET YOUR NEEDS

We're each unique, and most of us have needs and preferences that go beyond deciding when to schedule our practice sessions. If we want to create an exercise program that we can stick with over time, we have to meet the needs of our bodies. Let your body speak to you as you move toward restoring your flexibility. Would you like to add more energy to your program? Or are some of the sessions wearing you out? Does your body complain when you practice certain poses or sequences? Which poses and sequences feel especially good and natural to you?

The Restoring Flexibility four-week program is designed to be tweaked! Here are some tips for adapting the program to your personal needs and preferences.

- If you're past midlife and you've been fairly sedentary for a while, you may want to practice only sessions 1, 2, 3, and 4 during your first four-week program. Practice them in session order for your first two weeks, just as they're shown on the at-a-glance reference chart, and repeat them in session order for your second two weeks. This will allow you to get used to the sequences by practicing each of them more frequently, allow your body to adapt gradually to gentle exercise, and also allow you to practice every sequence in the Restoring Flexibility program except the Sun Salutation.

- No matter your age, if you're a former or current yoga practitioner and are familiar with the poses and sequences in *Restoring Flexibility*, you might try practicing only sessions 4, 5, 6, and 7 during your four-week program. Practice them in session order for your first two weeks, and repeat them in session order for your second two weeks. These are the four highest-energy practice sessions in the Restoring Flexibility program, so they offer a jump-start into a regular, ongoing yoga flexibility practice while allowing you to enjoy all eight sequences in the program.

- If you have health considerations that go beyond your bones and muscles, such as heart disease, cancer therapy, lung disease, or other non-musculoskeletal conditions, the practice sessions in the Restoring Flexibility program may, with approval from your doctor, offer you ways to gently stretch and move so that you can stay flexible and keep your joints and muscle fibers healthy. If you need extremely gentle practice sessions that won't raise your heart rate, keep you standing for too long, or leave you breathless, try practicing sessions 1, 8, 1, and 6 in that order. If the regular-length practice sessions are too much for you, try the morning, evening, or go-anywhere mini-sessions at whatever time of day you have the energy for them.

- No matter the state of your body, you might want to practice gentle yoga-based exercise more than twice a week. That's when the Restoring Flexibility mini-sessions can really come in handy. Practice your favorite mini anytime you feel like including 10 minutes of yoga-based flexibility exercise in your day.

- One of the greatest misconceptions about exercise is that if we don't have time to practice a full workout or session, we shouldn't bother. Nothing could be further from the truth. Anything is always better than nothing. For example, if you want to do something good for your body and only have three minutes, take off your shoes and socks and enjoy the Ankles, Feet, and Toes practice in Sequence 7. Your feet will thank you!

TWEAKING YOUR PROGRAM

After about three weeks, you'll have a pretty good idea of how well your program is serving you, both from a scheduling perspective and from your body's perspective. This is a good time to consider whether you want to tweak your program. Here are some questions to help you assess how well your yoga flexibility program is working for you. They'll bring you back to the three essential elements of a sustainable yoga flexibility practice: enjoyment of the practice itself, rightness for your body, and ease of scheduling.

ENJOYMENT OF YOUR PRACTICE AND RIGHTNESS FOR YOUR BODY

For each of the eight practice sequences, ask yourself these three questions:

- **How much do I enjoy this sequence?**

  Possible answers: 1) very much 2) maybe it will grow on me 3) not at all.

- **How easy or difficult does this sequence feel to me?**

  Possible answers: 1) easy 2) not easy, but not too difficult, either 3) difficult.

- **How well does this sequence meet my physical needs?**

  Possible answers: 1) very well 2) it will do for now 3) not well at all.

You probably won't stay with a program that feels like an uphill battle. At the same time, you'll reap the benefits of the Restoring Flexibility program more fully if you practice sequences that challenge you in ways that don't hurt and allow you to expand your comfort zone over time. Try to balance these considerations, keeping in mind that you're the one who knows what's best for you.

EASE OF SCHEDULING

Experts say that when you're trying to form a new habit, you should stick with it for about three weeks before giving up on it. And even then, they say, don't give up. Just assess and revise. These two questions are designed to help you do that.

Over the past three weeks:

- How many practice sessions have you missed? One? Two? More than two?

- How many times have you had to practice on a day or at a time other than the one on which you had originally planned? Once? Twice? More than twice?

If you've missed more than two practice sessions or you've found that you're often not able to practice when you had hoped, try some small tweaks in your schedule. If you can find a way to stay with your flexibility program for six or seven weeks in a row, you're more likely to stick with it long term. Remember, you can't change the direction of the wind, but you can always reset your sails!

APPENDICES

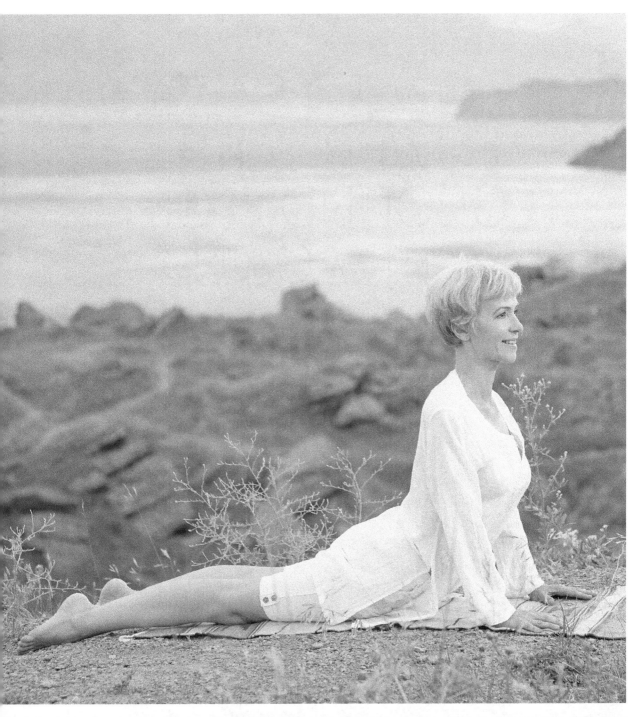

HOW TO SAFELY LOWER TO THE GROUND & GET UP AGAIN

The following four-part sequence shows how to comfortably lower to the ground and get up again while keeping your hips and shoulders in their natural, front-facing skeletal alignment. This method will help keep your low back safe as you move from a standing position to your hands and knees, from your hands and knees to a seated position on the ground, from a seated position back up to your hands and knees, and, finally, from your hands and knees up to a standing position.

Because we must resist gravity, rising is more difficult than lowering, so this appendix also shows how to use a chair for support when lowering to your hands and knees and rising from them. If you're uncertain about whether you can get up from the ground, make sure you have someone with you who can help in case you have trouble getting up, even if you're using a chair as a helper. Above all, please heed this advice: If you or those who know you best have concerns about whether you can safely rise from the ground, consult your doctor before trying to do so.

LOWERING TO YOUR HANDS AND KNEES FROM A STANDING POSITION

1. Begin in a standing position at the front of your mat. Make sure your feet are about hip-width apart.

2. From a standing position, gently hinge forward from your hip creases (the places where your legs meet your trunk), bending your knees as you bring your buttocks back and out.

   This gentle squat allows you to keep a long, straight back, rather than rounding from your waist as you bend.

3. Lower your arms, bringing your fingertips or fists down to the mat a few inches in front of your feet.

4. Bring your right foot way back behind your right arm.

5. Lower your right knee to the mat.

6. Bring your left knee back beside your right knee. Keep your knees about hip-width apart.

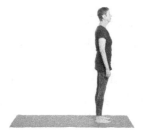

Begin in a standing position.

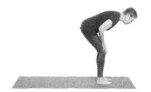

Gently fold forward.

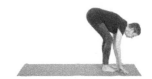

Lower arms.

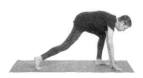

Bring right foot back.

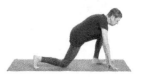

Lower right knee to mat.

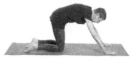

Bring left knee back.

LOWERING TO A SEATED POSITION FROM YOUR HANDS AND KNEES

1. Walk your knees toward the right so that your knees are under your hips. Keep your palms or fists on the mat.

2. Lower the outside of your left thigh to the mat. Rest your right thigh on or near your left thigh.

3. Swing your legs around to the left in order to sit facing forward on the mat.

4. Sit facing forward on your mat.

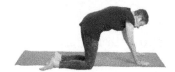

Walk knees toward right.

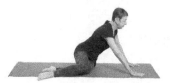

Lower left thigh to mat.

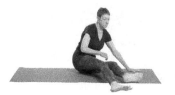

Swing legs around.

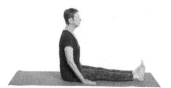

Face forward.

RISING TO YOUR HANDS AND KNEES FROM A SEATED POSITION

1. From a forward-facing seated position, bend your knees toward the right.

   Keep your arms facing forward as you bring your palms or fists to the mat.

2. Rise to your hands and knees by pressing your palms or fists into the mat and lifting your hips off the ground.

3. Walk your knees to the left so that your knees are under your hips.

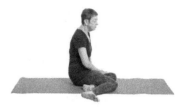

Bend knees toward right.

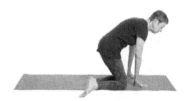

Rise to hands and knees.

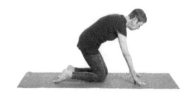

Walk knees to the left.

RISING TO A STANDING POSITION FROM YOUR HANDS AND KNEES

1. Bring your left foot forward toward your left hand. Now you're down on one knee.

2. Lift your right knee off the mat.

3. Walk your right foot forward, keeping your knees softly bent.

4. Rise halfway. Take a breath so that your blood pressure can adjust.

5. Slowly rise the rest of the way.

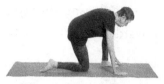

Bring left foot forward.

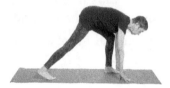

Lift right knee.

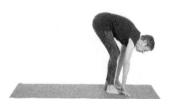

Walk right foot forward.

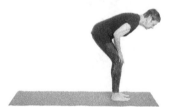

Rise halfway.

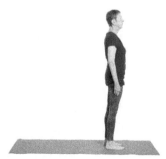

Rise to stand.

LOWERING TO YOUR HANDS AND KNEES USING A CHAIR FOR SUPPORT

1. Place a sturdy chair at the front of your yoga mat. Make sure that the front legs of the chair are on the mat. Stand one or two feet in front of the chair, as shown.

2. Fold forward from your hip creases, gently bending your knees as you bring your buttocks back and out. Place your hands firmly on the sides of the chair seat.

3. Bring your right foot way back behind your right arm and come to your right toes.

4. Lower your right knee to the mat.

5. Lower your left knee down beside your right knee. Keep your knees about hip-width apart.

6. Bring your palms or fists to the mat. You're now on your hands and knees.

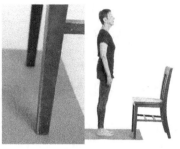

Face chair.

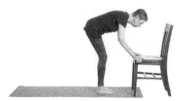

Place hands firmly on chair seat.

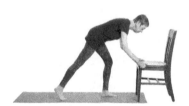

Bring right foot back.

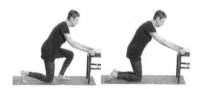

Lower right knee. Bring left knee down beside right knee.

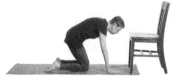

Bring hands to mat.

RISING FROM YOUR HANDS AND KNEES USING A CHAIR FOR SUPPORT

1. From your hands and knees, rise to your knees and place your hands on the chair seat, just as you did when you lowered.

2. Bring your left foot forward, closer to the chair.

3. Lift your right knee up off the mat and come to your right toes.

4. Walk your right foot forward.

5. Gently rise to a standing position.

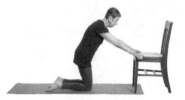

Place hands firmly on chair seat.

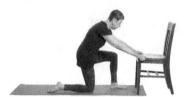

Bring left foot forward.

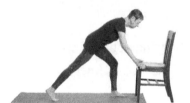

Lift right knee up off mat.

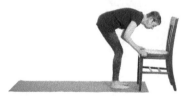

Walk right foot forward.

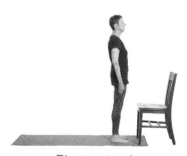

Rise to stand.

SESSION GUIDES

Each guide shows the numbered steps for all practice sequences in that session, exactly as they are shown in each sequence's chapter in *Restoring Flexibility*. Each guide has been designed to fit on two pages that face each other, so you can lay the book out flat, see all the poses and sequences for one session at a glance, and read the names of the poses easily, even when the book is on the floor or on a nearby table or countertop.

Keep your guide handy as you practice. It will help you remember each sequence's component poses so you won't need to keep referring back to each separate book chapter. This will make it easier to keep your focus as you practice and make your practice even more refreshing.

RESTORING FLEXIBILITY
GUIDE TO SESSION 1

WEEK 1, DAY 1 OF THE FOUR-WEEK PROGRAM

ALIGNING YOUR BONES/CENTERING YOUR BREATH

1. Ground and Grow into Mountain Pose

2. Breathe in Stillness

3. Move with Your Breath: Namaste Circles

4. Return to Mountain Pose

RESTORING UPPER BODY FLEXIBILITY

1. Mountain Pose

2. Gentle Neck Twist

3. Arm Circles

4. Bent-Elbow Chest and Back Stretch

5. Standing Side Bend

6. Standing Twist

7. Return to Mountain Pose

8. Repeat the Sequence Once

RESTORING LOWER BODY FLEXIBILITY

1. Staff Pose
2. Optional: Exercise Ankles, Feet, Toes
3. Wide-Leg Forward Fold
4. Head Toward Knee, Right Knee Bent
5. Revolved Head Toward Knee, Right Knee Bent
6. Repeat Wide-Leg Forward Fold
7. Head Toward Knee, Left Knee Bent
8. Revolved Head Toward Knee, Left Knee Bent
9. Bound Angle Pose
10. Return to Staff Pose

RECLINING JOINT RELEASES/MUSCLE RELAXATION

1. Lower to Back
2. Full-Body Stretch (twice)
3. Reclining Bent-Knee Twist with Arm Extension, Knees Facing Left
4. Reclining Bent-Knee Twist with Arm Extension, Knees Facing Right
5. Knees Toward Chest (twice)
6. Reclining Bound Angle
7. Full-Body Stretch (twice)
8. Optional: Savasana

OPTIONAL: ANKLES, FEET, & TOES FLEXIBILITY SEQUENCE

1. Rotate ankles
2. Wiggle toes
3. Curl toes
4. Spread toes
5. Point toes strongly away from ankles
6. Point toes strongly toward ankles
7. Bring soles of feet closer to each other
8. Move soles of feet farther from each other

RESTORING FLEXIBILITY
GUIDE TO SESSION 2

WEEK 1, DAY 2 OF THE FOUR-WEEK PROGRAM

ALIGNING YOUR BONES/CENTERING YOUR BREATH

1. Ground and Grow into Mountain Pose
2. Breathe in Stillness
3. Move with Your Breath: Namaste Circles
4. Return to Mountain Pose

RESTORING UPPER BODY FLEXIBILITY

1. Mountain Pose
2. Gentle Neck Twist
3. Arm Circles
4. Bent-Elbow Chest and Back Stretch
5. Standing Side Bend
6. Standing Twist
7. Return to Mountain Pose
8. Repeat the Sequence Once

RESTORING HIP FLEXIBILITY—FLEXORS

1. Extended-Leg Stance, Left Leg Back
2. Warrior I, Right Knee Bent
3. One-Sided Stretch with Forearms on Back, Left Leg Back
4. Repeat Warrior I, Right Knee Bent
5. One-Sided Stretch with Twist and Arm Opening, Left Leg Back
6. Return to Mountain Pose
7. Extended-Leg Stance, Right Leg Back
8. Warrior I, Left Knee Bent
9. One-Sided Stretch with Forearms on Back, Right Leg Back
10. Repeat Warrior I, Left Knee Bent
11. One-Sided Stretch with Twist and Arm Opening, Right Leg Back
12. Return to Mountain Pose

RESTORING LOWER BODY FLEXIBILITY

1. Staff Pose
2. Optional: Exercise Ankles, Feet, Toes
3. Wide-Leg Forward Fold
4. Head Toward Knee, Right Knee Bent
5. Revolved Head Toward Knee, Right Knee Bent
6. Repeat Wide-Leg Forward Fold
7. Head Toward Knee, Left Knee Bent
8. Revolved Head Toward Knee, Left Knee Bent
9. Bound Angle Pose
10. Return to Staff Pose

OPTIONAL: ANKLES, FEET, & TOES FLEXIBILITY SEQUENCE

1. Rotate ankles
2. Wiggle toes
3. Curl toes
4. Spread toes
5. Point toes strongly away from ankles
6. Point toes strongly toward ankles
7. Bring soles of feet closer to each other
8. Move soles of feet farther from each other

RESTORING FLEXIBILITY
GUIDE TO SESSION 3

WEEK 2, DAY 1 OF THE FOUR-WEEK PROGRAM

ALIGNING YOUR BONES/CENTERING YOUR BREATH

1. Ground and Grow into Mountain Pose

2. Breathe in Stillness

3. Move with Your Breath: Namaste Circles

4. Return to Mountain Pose

RESTORING SPINAL FLEXIBILITY

1. Tabletop Pose

2. Cat/Cow Spinal Flexibility Flow

3. Extended Puppy Pose

4. Threading the Needle with Optional Arm Raise, Left Arm Threaded

5. Return to Tabletop

6. Threading the Needle with Optional Arm Raise, Right Arm Threaded

7. Repeat Extended Puppy Pose

8. Camel Pose

9. Return to Tabletop

RESTORING HIP FLEXIBILITY—ROTATORS, ADDUCTORS, ABDUCTORS

1. Wide-Leg Stance

2. Triangle Pose, Left Foot Turned Out

3. Side Angle Pose with Optional Arm Extension, Left Knee Bent

4. Repeat Triangle Pose, Left Leg Turned Out

5. Return to Wide-Leg Stance

6. Wide-Leg Forward Fold with Twist and Left Arm Opening

7. Wide-Leg Forward Fold with Twist and Right Arm Opening

8. Triangle Pose, Right Leg Turned Out

9. Side Angle Pose and Optional Arm Extension, Right Knee Bent

10. Repeat Triangle Pose, Right Leg Turned Out

11. Return to Wide-Leg Stance

RECLINING JOINT RELEASES/MUSCLE RELAXATION

1. Lower to Back

2. Full-Body Stretch (twice)

3. Reclining Bent-Knee Twist with Arm Extension, Knees Facing Left

4. Reclining Bent-Knee Twist with Arm Extension, Knees Facing Right

5. Knees Toward Chest (twice)

6. Reclining Bound Angle

7. Full-Body Stretch (twice)

8. Optional: Savasana

RESTORING FLEXIBILITY
GUIDE TO SESSION 4

ALIGNING YOUR BONES/CENTERING YOUR BREATH

1. Ground and Grow into Mountain Pose
2. Breathe in Stillness
3. Move with Your Breath: Namaste Circles
4. Return to Mountain Pose

RESTORING SPINAL FLEXIBILITY

1. Tabletop Pose
2. Cat/Cow Spinal Flexibility Flow
3. Extended Puppy Pose
4. Threading the Needle with Optional Arm Raise, Left Arm Threaded
5. Return to Tabletop
6. Threading the Needle with Optional Arm Raise, Right Arm Threaded
7. Repeat Extended Puppy Pose
8. Camel Pose
9. Return to Tabletop

RESTORING HIP FLEXIBILITY—FLEXORS

1. Extended-Leg Stance, Left Leg Back
2. Warrior I, Right Knee Bent
3. One-Sided Stretch with Forearms on Back, Left Leg Back
4. Repeat Warrior I, Right Knee Bent
5. One-Sided Stretch with Twist and Arm Opening, Left Leg Back
6. Return to Mountain Pose
7. Extended-Leg Stance, Right Leg Back
8. Warrior I, Left Knee Bent
9. One-Sided Stretch with Forearms on Back, Right Leg Back
10. Repeat Warrior I, Left Knee Bent

11. One-Sided Stretch with Twist and Arm Opening, Right Leg Back

12. Return to Mountain Pose

RESTORING LOWER BODY FLEXIBILITY

1. Staff Pose

2. Optional: Exercise Ankles, Feet, Toes

3. Wide-Leg Forward Fold

4. Head Toward Knee, Right Knee Bent

5. Revolved Head Toward Knee, Right Knee Bent

6. Repeat Wide-Leg Forward Fold

7. Head Toward Knee, Left Knee Bent

8. Revolved Head Toward Knee, Left Knee Bent

9. Bound Angle Pose

10. Return to Staff Pose

OPTIONAL: ANKLES, FEET, & TOES FLEXIBILITY SEQUENCE

1. Rotate ankles

2. Wiggle toes

3. Curl toes

4. Spread toes

5. Point toes strongly away from ankles

6. Point toes strongly toward ankles

7. Bring soles of feet closer to each other

8. Move soles of feet farther from each other

RESTORING FLEXIBILITY
GUIDE TO SESSION 5

WEEK 3, DAY 1 OF THE FOUR-WEEK PROGRAM

ALIGNING YOUR BONES/CENTERING YOUR BREATH

1. Ground and Grow into Mountain Pose

2. Breathe in Stillness

3. Move with Your Breath: Namaste Circles

4. Return to Mountain Pose

RESTORING UPPER BODY FLEXIBILITY

1. Mountain Pose

2. Gentle Neck Twist

3. Arm Circles

4. Bent-Elbow Chest and Back Stretch

5. Standing Side Bend

6. Standing Twist

7. Return to Mountain Pose

8. Repeat the Sequence Once

THE YOGA SUN SALUTATION

1. Upward Salute

2. Forward Fold

3. Low Lunge, Left Leg Back

4. Low Plank

5. Lower to Belly

6. Low Cobra

7. Rise to Low Plank

8. Downward-Facing Dog

9. Rise to Forward Fold

10. Rise to Upward Salute

11. Repeat the entire sequence, this time bringing your right leg back for Low Lunge

RECLINING JOINT RELEASES/MUSCLE RELAXATION

1. Lower to Back

2. Full-Body Stretch (twice)

3. Reclining Bent-Knee Twist with Arm Extension, Knees Facing Left

4. Reclining Bent-Knee Twist with Arm Extension, Knees Facing Right

5. Knees Toward Chest (twice)

6. Reclining Bound Angle

7. Full-Body Stretch (twice)

8. Optional: Savasana

RESTORING FLEXIBILITY
GUIDE TO SESSION 6

ALIGNING YOUR BONES/CENTERING YOUR BREATH

1. Ground and Grow into Mountain Pose

2. Breathe in Stillness

3. Move with Your Breath: Namaste Circles

4. Return to Mountain Pose

RESTORING HIP FLEXIBILITY: ROTATORS, ADDUCTORS, ABDUCTORS

1. Wide-Leg Stance

2. Triangle Pose, Left Foot Turned Out

3. Side Angle Pose with Optional Arm Extension, Left Knee Bent

4. Repeat Triangle Pose, Left Leg Turned Out

5. Return to Wide-Leg Stance

6. Wide-Leg Forward Fold with Twist and Left Arm Opening

7. Wide-Leg Forward Fold with Twist and Right Arm Opening

8. Triangle Pose, Right Leg Turned Out

9. Side Angle Pose and Optional Arm Extension, Right Knee Bent

10. Repeat Triangle Pose, Right Leg Turned Out

11. Return to Wide-Leg Stance

RESTORING LOWER BODY FLEXIBILITY

1. Staff Pose

2. Wide-Leg Forward Fold

3. Head Toward Knee, Right Knee Bent

4. Revolved Head Toward Knee, Right Knee Bent

5. Repeat Wide-Leg Forward Fold

6. Head Toward Knee, Left Knee Bent

7. Revolved Head Toward Knee, Left Knee Bent

8. Bound Angle Pose

9. Return to Staff Pose

RECLINING JOINT RELEASES/MUSCLE RELAXATION

1. Lower to Back

2. Full-Body Stretch (twice)

3. Reclining Bent-Knee Twist with Arm Extension, Knees Facing Left

4. Reclining Bent-Knee Twist with Arm Extension, Knees Facing Right

5. Knees Toward Chest (twice)

6. Reclining Bound Angle

7. Full-Body Stretch (twice)

8. Optional: Savasana

RESTORING FLEXIBILITY
GUIDE TO SESSION 7

WEEK 4, DAY 1 OF THE FOUR-WEEK PROGRAM

ALIGNING YOUR BONES/CENTERING YOUR BREATH

1. Ground and Grow into Mountain Pose

2. Breathe in Stillness

3. Move with Your Breath: Namaste Circles

4. Return to Mountain Pose

RESTORING SPINAL FLEXIBILITY

1. Tabletop Pose

2. Cat/Cow Spinal Flexibility Flow

3. Extended Puppy Pose

4. Threading the Needle with Optional Arm Raise, Left Arm Threaded

5. Return to Tabletop

6. Threading the Needle with Optional Arm Raise, Right Arm Threaded

7. Repeat Extended Puppy Pose

8. Camel Pose

9. Return to Tabletop

THE YOGA SUN SALUTATION

1. Upward Salute

2. Forward Fold

3. Low Lunge, Left Leg Back

4. Low Plank

5. Lower to Belly

6. Low Cobra

7. Rise to Low Plank

8. Downward-Facing Dog

9. Rise to Forward Fold

10. Rise to Upward Salute

11. Repeat the entire sequence, this time bringing your right leg back for Low Lunge

RECLINING JOINT RELEASES/MUSCLE RELAXATION

1. Lower to Back

2. Full-Body Stretch (twice)

3. Reclining Bent-Knee Twist with Arm Extension, Knees Facing Left

4. Reclining Bent-Knee Twist with Arm Extension, Knees Facing Right

5. Knees Toward Chest (twice)

6. Reclining Bound Angle

7. Full-Body Stretch (twice)

8. Optional: Savasana

RESTORING FLEXIBILITY
GUIDE TO SESSION 8

WEEK 4, DAY 2 OF THE FOUR-WEEK PROGRAM

ALIGNING YOUR BONES/CENTERING YOUR BREATH

1. Ground and Grow into Mountain Pose

2. Breathe in Stillness

3. Move with Your Breath: Namaste Circles

4. Return to Mountain Pose

RESTORING UPPER BODY FLEXIBILITY

1. Mountain Pose

2. Gentle Neck Twist

3. Arm Circles

4. Bent-Elbow Chest and Back Stretch

5. Standing Side Bend

6. Standing Twist

7. Return to Mountain Pose

8. Repeat the Sequence Once

RESTORING HIP FLEXIBILITY: ROTATORS, ADDUCTORS, ABDUCTORS

1. Wide-Leg Stance

2. Triangle Pose, Left Foot Turned Out

3. Side Angle Pose with Optional Arm Extension, Left Knee Bent

4. Repeat Triangle Pose, Left Leg Turned Out

5. Return to Wide-Leg Stance

6. Wide-Leg Forward Fold with Twist and Left Arm Opening

7. Wide-Leg Forward Fold with Twist and Right Arm Opening

8. Triangle Pose, Right Leg Turned Out

9. Side Angle Pose and Optional Arm Extension, Right Knee Bent

10. Repeat Triangle Pose, Right Leg Turned Out

11. Return to Wide-Leg Stance

RESTORING LOWER BODY FLEXIBILITY

1. Staff Pose

2. Optional: Exercise Ankles, Feet, Toes

3. Wide-Leg Forward Fold

4. Head Toward Knee, Right Knee Bent

5. Revolved Head Toward Knee, Right Knee Bent

6. Repeat Wide-Leg Forward Fold

7. Head Toward Knee, Left Knee Bent

8. Revolved Head Toward Knee, Left Knee Bent

9. Bound Angle Pose

10. Return to Staff Pose

OPTIONAL: ANKLES, FEET, & TOES FLEXIBILITY SEQUENCE

1. Rotate ankles

2. Wiggle toes

3. Curl toes

4. Spread toes

5. Point toes strongly away from ankles

6. Point toes strongly toward ankles

7. Bring soles of feet closer to each other

8. Move soles of feet farther from each other

RESTORING FLEXIBILITY
GUIDE TO MORNING MINI-SESSION

RESTORING UPPER BODY FLEXIBILITY

1. Mountain Pose

2. Gentle Neck Twist

3. Arm Circles

4. Bent-Elbow Chest and Back Stretch

5. Standing Side Bend

6. Standing Twist

7. Return to Mountain Pose

8. Repeat the Sequence Once

RESTORING LOWER BODY FLEXIBILITY

1. Staff Pose

2. Optional: Exercise Ankles, Feet, Toes

3. Wide-Leg Forward Fold

4. Head Toward Knee, Right Knee Bent

5. Revolved Head Toward Knee, Right Knee Bent

6. Repeat Wide-Leg Forward Fold

7. Head Toward Knee, Left Knee Bent

8. Revolved Head Toward Knee, Left Knee Bent

9. Bound Angle Pose

10. Rise

OPTIONAL: ANKLES, FEET, & TOES
FLEXIBILITY SEQUENCE

1. Rotate ankles

2. Wiggle toes

3. Curl toes

4. Spread toes

5. Point toes strongly away from ankles

6. Point toes strongly toward ankles

7. Bring soles of feet closer to each other

8. Move soles of feet farther from each other

RESTORING FLEXIBILITY
GUIDE TO MIDDAY MINI-SESSION

ALIGNING YOUR BONES/CENTERING YOUR BREATH

1. Ground and Grow into Mountain Pose

2. Breathe in Stillness

3. Move with Your Breath: Namaste Circles

4. Return to Mountain Pose

THE YOGA SUN SALUTATION

1. Upward Salute

2. Forward Fold

3. Low Lunge, Left Leg Back

4. Low Plank

5. Lower to Belly

6. Low Cobra

7. Rise to Low Plank

8. Downward-Facing Dog

9. Rise to Forward Fold

10. Rise to Upward Salute

11. Repeat the entire sequence, this time bringing your right leg back for Low Lunge

RESTORING FLEXIBILITY
GUIDE TO EVENING MINI-SESSION

RESTORING LOWER BODY FLEXIBILITY

1. Staff Pose

2. Wide-Leg Forward Fold

3. Head Toward Knee, Right Knee Bent

4. Revolved Head Toward Knee, Right Knee Bent

5. Repeat Wide-Leg Forward Fold

6. Head Toward Knee, Left Knee Bent

7. Revolved Head Toward Knee, Left Knee Bent

8. Bound Angle Pose

9. Lower to Back and Recline

RECLINING JOINT RELEASES/MUSCLE RELAXATION

1. Lower to Back

2. Full-Body Stretch (twice)

3. Reclining Bent-Knee Twist with Arm Extension, Knees Facing Left

4. Reclining Bent-Knee Twist with Arm Extension, Knees Facing Right

5. Knees Toward Chest (twice)

6. Reclining Bound Angle

7. Full-Body Stretch (twice)

8. Optional: Savasana

RESTORING FLEXIBILITY
GUIDE TO GO-ANYWHERE MINI-SESSION

ALIGNING YOUR BONES/CENTERING YOUR BREATH

1. Ground and Grow into Mountain Pose

2. Breathe in Stillness

3. Move with Your Breath: Namaste Circles

4. Return to Mountain Pose

RESTORING UPPER BODY FLEXIBILITY

1. Mountain Pose

2. Gentle Neck Twist

3. Arm Circles

4. Bent-Elbow Chest and Back Stretch

5. Standing Side Bend

6. Standing Twist

7. Return to Mountain Pose

8. Repeat the Sequence Once

NOTES

1. Robert Butler, *The Longevity Revolution* (New York: PublicAffairs, 2008), xi.

2. "Calculators: Life Expectancy," *Social Security*, accessed January 2015, www.ssa.gov/planners/lifeexpectancy.html.

3. Harvard School of Public Health, "Strength and Flexibility Training," *Nutrition Source*, accessed December 14, 2014, www.hsph.harvard.edu/nutritionsource/strength-and-flexibility-training.

4. C. J. Brown and K. L. Flood, "Mobility Limitation in the Older Patient: A Clinical Review," *Journal of the American Medical Association* 310, no. 11 (September 18, 2013): 1169.

5. Ibid., 1175.

6. S. G. Wannamethee et al., "From a Postal Questionnaire of Older Men, Healthy Lifestyle Factors Reduced the Onset of and May Have Increased Recovery from Mobility Limitation," *Journal of Clinical Epidemiology* 58, no. 8 (June 14, 2005), www.jclinepi.com/article/S0895-4356(05)00090-9/abstract.

7. European Society of Cardiology Press Office, "Ability to Sit and Rise from the Floor Is Closely Correlated with All-Cause Mortality Rate," *European Society of Cardiology*, published December 13, 2012, www.escardio.org/The-ESC/Press-Office/Press-releases/Last-5-years/Ability-to-sit-and-rise-from-the-floor-is-closely-correlated-with-all-cause-mort. This press release references the following scholarly article: L. B. Brito et al.,

"Ability to Sit and Rise from the Floor as a Predictor of All-Cause Mortality," *European Journal of Cardiovascular Prevention* 21, no. 7 (November 29, 2012): 892-93.

8. Ibid.

9. Gretchen Reynolds, "How Exercise Keeps Us Young," *New York Times*, January 7, 2015, http://well.blogs.nytimes.com/2015/01/07/how-exercise-keeps-us-young.

10. Gretchen Reynolds, "Aging Well Through Exercise," *New York Times*, November 9, 2011, http://well.blogs.nytimes.com/2011/11/09/aging-well-through-exercise.

11. Paula Chu et al., "The Effectiveness of Yoga in Modifying Risk Factors for Cardiovascular Disease and Metabolic Syndrome," *European Journal of Preventative Cardiology* (December 14, 2014): 14.

12. Kimberlee B. Bonura, "The Psychological Benefits of Yoga Practice for Older Adults: Evidence and Guidelines," *International Journal of Yoga Therapy*, No. 21 (2011): 131.

13. Steffany Haaz, "Yoga for Arthritis," *Johns Hopkins Arthritis Center*, published June 23, 2009, www.hopkinsarthritis.org/patient-corner/disease-management/yoga-for-arthritis.

14. McKinley Health Center, *Neck Pain*, University of Illinois at Urbana-Champaign, HEd. 11-105, January 19, 2010.

INDEX

ACKNOWLEDGMENTS

This book would not have been possible without my magnificent yoga students. They, more than any formal training I've taken, have been my teachers. I want to especially thank my longtime students at the West 7th Community Center in St. Paul, Minnesota, including—but certainly not limited to—Marva Bohen, Anne Butler, Chuck Butler, Judy Ewald, Julia Fish, Carole Heimdahl, Claudia Munson, Margaret Sebaka, Mike Sebaka, Pam Scinocca, Linda Slattengren, Jackie Trucker, Connie Warner, and Leon Webster. These brilliant and generous yoga practitioners reviewed—and corrected, bless you!—all the practice sequences in *Restoring Flexibility*. Thank you, one and all.

Thank you, too, to the generous staff at West 7th Community Center (Debbie, Jeannie, Marilee, and Teisha), and to the gentle gentlemen who make sure that our classroom is shipshape.

I want to thank another of my beloved yoga students, publishing consultant Laurie Harper of Author Biz Consulting, for helping me bring this book to publication. It was Laurie's astute advice and guidance, along with her genuine belief in the value of my approach to teaching yoga to older adults, that opened the door to publication. Thank you, Laurie.

I'm deeply indebted to my community-based University of Minnesota colleagues, psychologist Donna Bennett and family practice physician Bill Spinelli, for their work on developing practical, meaningful programs on positive aging for baby boomers. It was their work that raised my consciousness and helped me formulate ways to help meet the need for age-appropriate, body-sensitive yoga-based exercise for people in midlife and beyond. Thank you, Bill and Donna.

I also want to thank Judy Gilats for reading *Restoring Flexibility* with her keen literary eye. Thank you, Judy.

Finally, my heartfelt thanks to Ulysses Press for their commitment to helping our country's 60 million seniors stay physically fit, active, and independent. Thank you to acquisitions editor Casie Vogel and to editors Claire Chun and Lily Chou for your amazingly insightful help every step of the way, and thank you to our masterful, engaging models, yoga instructor Baxter Bell and personal trainer Toni Silver.

ABOUT THE AUTHOR

Andrea Gilats, PhD, RYT, is a certified yoga teacher, writer, and nationally recognized expert on later-life learning who spent three decades as an award-winning educational leader at the University of Minnesota. Through Third Age Yoga, her community-based teaching practice, she has worked with hundreds of vital people in their 50s, 60s, 70s, and beyond who seek a body-sensitive, age-appropriate approach to yoga. Her Third Age Yoga videos have been viewed over 20,000 times on YouTube, and she offers helpful tidbits about yoga, exercise, and aging well on her Third Age Yoga Facebook page. Visit thirdageyoga.net for information about her classes.

Printed in the USA
CPSIA information can be obtained
at www.ICGtesting.com
LVHW061048050923
757272LV00013B/1091